SURGERY - PROCEDURES, COMPLICATIONS, AND RESULTS

ANASTOMOSES

TYPES, TECHNIQUES/PROCEDURES, CLINICAL OUTCOMES AND COMPLICATIONS

SURGERY - PROCEDURES, COMPLICATIONS, AND RESULTS

Additional books in this series can be found on Nova's website under the Series tab.

Additional e-books in this series can be found on Nova's website under the e-book tab.

SURGERY - PROCEDURES, COMPLICATIONS, AND RESULTS

ANASTOMOSES

TYPES, TECHNIQUES/PROCEDURES, CLINICAL OUTCOMES AND COMPLICATIONS

FRANCES C. KING
AND
MCKINLEY A. MALLOY
EDITORS

NOVA BIOMEDICAL

New York

For permission to use material from this book please contact us:
Telephone 631-231-7269; Fax 631-231-8175
Web Site: http://www.novapublishers.com

Additional color graphics may be available in the e-book version of this book.

Library of Congress Cataloging-in-Publication Data

ISBN: 978-1-62618-657-6

Library of Congress Control Number: 2013935913

Published by Nova Science Publishers, Inc. † New York

Contents

Preface

In this book, the authors present current research in the study of the types, techniques/procedures, clinical outcomes and complications of surgical anastomoses. Topics discussed include bilioenteric anastomoses; intestinal anastomosis education and training; invaginating colonic anastomosis; expandable devices for easier, quicker and more efficient aortic-prosthesis anastomosis; and potential postoperative complications associated with bowel anastomosis.

Chapter I – Bilioenteric anastomoses (BEA) are a frequent surgical procedure performed under different scenarios. The main objective of BEA is to allow adequate bile outflow into the gastrointestinal tract and prevent future biliary strictures that will compromise adequate bile drainage, leading to repeated episodes of cholangitis, secondary biliary cirrhosis and death. Indications for this procedure include benign diseases (strictures of the biliary tract, iatrogenic bile duct injuries, choledochal cysts) and malignant diseases (pancreatic cancer and distal cholangiocarcinoma). Since Winiwaters' first description of a bilioenteric reconstruction more than 100 years ago, major technical advances have occurred through time. Bilioenteric anastomoses can be classified as extra-hepatic and intra-hepatic, depending of the anatomical area of the biliary tract used. Extra-hepatic anastomoses include choledochoduodenostomy, choledochojejunostomy, and hepatojejunostomy. Intra-hepatic anastomoses include hepaticojejunostomy (Hepp-Couinaud) and peripheral cholangiojejunostomy (Longmire-Sanford). The Hepp-Couinaud technique is the most frequently performed anastomosis. This approach exposes the extra-hepatic course of the left hepatic duct and allows a wide anastomosis to a Roux-en-Y jejunal loop. The use of trans-anastomotic stents is no longer necessary and has limited indications. Complications of BEA include cholangitis, biliary fistula, intra-abdominal abscesses and strictures. Long-term follow-up report excellent results in 90% of the patients. Sixty-five percent of recurrent strictures develop during the first 2 years and 80% during the first 5- years after surgery. In this chapter the authors present the most frequently BEA techniques performed, their complications and outcome.

Chapter II – The aim of a gastro-intestinal suture is to provide a hermetic closure in the intestine or in an anastomosis.

To achieve a successful suture, a proper technique is essential, with strict adherence to surgical principles, such as suture tension, border vascularization and intestinal diameter. Also the patient biological condition has to be considered. All of these factors influence suture healing but the experience and skill of the surgeon are probably most important in the final outcome of the anastomosis.

Until recently the learning of any surgical procedure was based on direct operation on the patient, with initial supervision by an experienced surgeon. This has several drawbacks such as risks for the patient, long learning curves and an increase in operating room costs because of greater operation times. Laparoscopic procedures need even longer and more complex training periods due to the lack of tactile sensation and two-dimension view. The problem is even greater in the case of residents who are less experienced in surgery in general. To speed up learning and avoid direct training on patients, training laboratories have been designed, where physical and virtual reality simulators can be used.

The usefulness of training using simulation in basic surgical techniques has been shown in improving general surgical skills and performance of intestinal anastomosis with synthetic materials. Training in intestinal anastomosis using dead animal viscera is very similar to the clinical setting and has advantages over other options such as live animals, simulators or corpses. The training on live animals reproduces real clinical settings although it has drawbacks such as high costs or the sacrifice of the animal. Cadaver surgery is also very similar to real clinical settings but is hardly available. Virtual reality is very different from real clinical settings and evidence for validation of most designed devices is lacking. These models could be used as the first contact with laparoscopic training, according to the conclusions of the systematic reviews published to date. However, the advantage in resident training with some laparoscopic experience has not been shown. On the other hand these systems are expensive, although less so than direct training on patients.

As a result, the aim of this work is to expose which is the best training method in every anastomosis type and the influence that the different simulators or training with animals have on learning surgical skills.

Chapter III – The earliest reports of surgical suture date back to 3000 BC in ancient Egypt, and the oldest known suture is in a mummy from 1100 BC. The ancient Egyptians and Babylonians and the later Greeks and Romans used the intestines of herbivorous animals for much the same purposes. Detailed records of sigmoid volvulus were found in the Egyptian Papyrus Ebers and in ancient Greek and Roman writings. The ancient Egyptian Ebers papyrus describes the natural history of sigmoid volvulus as either reducing spontaneously, or the sigmoid colon being 'rotted'. Written in 500 BCE, the detailed description of a wound suture and the suture materials used in it is by the Indian sage and physician Sushruta.

Early in the first century AD, Celsus recorded attempts to suture the intestine but and Abulkasem in 87 AD, recommended using the jaws of large ants to unite intestinal wounds and referred to catgut made from the intestines of sheep as suture material. Other ancient surgical methods involved the use of a few large-diameter sutures; use of bone, trachea, or wood stents; or attempt to invaginate the cut ends of intestine. The oldest reported intestinal suturing technique is the Glover's suture that was a simple continuous stitch in which the ends, instead of being tied, were left long and pulled externally through the abdominal wound.

Chapter IV – Open thoracic aorta prosthetic substitution still carries significant mortality and serious complications risk, in particular to CNS. Risk is mostly correlated to the length of clamping/circulatory arrest time, i.e. essentially to the time required for vascular anastomosis construction.

We developed devices for easier, quicker and more efficient aortic-prosthesis anastomosis based on a new working principle: i.e. compression of vascular stump between inner (nitinol wireframe) and outer structures (external ligature or nitinol wireframe) instead of sewing with full-thickness perforation of the vessel wall.

The device consists of loops of nitinol wires, wrapped within a Dacron fabric and connected to a prosthesis end (Type I and III). The nitinol wire loops can be expanded and tightened by activating a removable guide in such a way that device varies its diameter, while maintaining a regular cylindrical shape. This allows the easy and quick insertion of the retracted device into the vascular stump and then its expansion to perfectly fit with the vessel diameter. Haemostasis and permanent device fixation are provided by external ligature/suture.

Three main models (Type I, II and III) applying the same working mechanism, but with different configurations, allow to fit with all aorta segments as well as special conditions of use.

Device type I, previously connected with a tube graft end, is used for the first anastomosis, either proximal or distal; device type II is then used for the second anastomosis after having tailored the graft tube at its appropriate length.

Device type III is ideally used for anastomosis in dissection cases, allowing in particular to include even the concavity of arch. Single graft layer type I devices for small diameters (6-14 mm) can be used for supraortic trunks.

The regularly expandable configuration of the ring device allows to solve all the insertion, positioning and stability problems of the 70ies intraluminal prosthesis. That makes performing anastomosis a very simple task, which can be carried out in seconds vs the 10-15 min per anastomosis at best required with hand suture.

The aortic wall being not perforated by the suture, the coupling is immediately blood-thigh ("air-tight" in fact!) and then independent by the integrity of the physiological coagulation mechanisms.

In summary favorable effects on complications rate, particularly in aortic arch substitution, related to circulatory arrest, hypothermia and CNS perfusion and dissection layers reconstructions can be expected due to:

1. dramatic reduction of the time required for completing aortic prosthetic anastomosis because of a) great simplification of anastomosis technique, which is performed at once with b) double strip graft vascular stump buttressing and c)"air-tight" sealing dissection layers re-approximation
2. easy and quick supraortic trunks anastomosis previously prepared on the main tube graft.

Anastomosis immediate blood-tightness not dependent on coagulation integrity may predictably decrease intra- and postoperative blood losses. Use of these devices may also enhance mininvasive access in prosthetic open substitution of any aortic segments.

Chapter V – Despite development of improved surgical techniques, advances in perioperative and critical care and introduction of broad-spectrum antibiotics, colorectal surgery continues to present with as a great challenge. Postoperative complications are common, occurring in 18-57% of patients after elective surgery and in 39.3-72% after emergency one. Potential postoperative complications associated with the colorrectal surgery are complications related to anastomosis.

There is nothing that provokes greater anxiety and consternation to the gastrointestinal surgeon than the prospect of a leak from a colonic or colorectal anastomosis. The consequences to the patient from such a complication can be significant and not infrequently life-threatening. A surgeon can only control some of the many variables in anastomotic construction. The fundamental principles of preservation of an adequate blood supply, total absence of tension on the suture line and healthy bowel for both the proximal and distal ends without thickening or inflammation have remained constant. The necessity of bowel preparation is now a topic of considerable debate, defending many surgeons not to be performed. The technical requirements include the creation of an airtight suture line, in some circumstances protected by a proximal diverting procedure, and/or omental wrap. Whether the anastomosis is hand-sewn in one or two layers, performed with interrupted or running suture technique, or constructed with a stapling device has no impact on leak rates. Factors often beyond the surgeon's control are immutable comorbidities and the patient's body habitus.

A safe anastomosis should include: not leak, cause no persistent bleeding, cause no stricture of the lumen and create no risk for internal hernia. An ideal anastomosis must be also easy to construct, consistently reproducible, and easy to teach.

The aim of paper is to review types, techniques, procedures, clinical outcomes and complications of colorectal anastomoses, including mechanical and hand-sewn sutures, of the colonic and colorectal anastomoses. The authors expect to help surgeons and surgical fellows to learn about this topic with particular attention to the risk factors and procedure-related complications.

In: Anastomoses ISBN: 978-1-62618-657-6
Editors: F. King, McKineley A. Malloy © 2013 Nova Science Publishers, Inc.

Chapter I

Bilioenteric Anastomoses

***Miguel Ángel Mercado*[*]**
***and Julio Alfaro Varela*[†]**
Department of Surgery, Instituto Nacional de Ciencias Médicas y Nutrición "Salvador Zubirán",
México City, México

Abstract

Bilioenteric anastomoses (BEA) are a frequent surgical procedure performed under different scenarios. The main objective of BEA is to allow adequate bile outflow into the gastrointestinal tract and prevent future biliary strictures that will compromise adequate bile drainage, leading to repeated episodes of cholangitis, secondary biliary cirrhosis and death. Indications for this procedure include benign diseases (strictures of the biliary tract, iatrogenic bile duct injuries, choledochal cysts) and malignant diseases (pancreatic cancer and distal cholangiocarcinoma). Since Winiwaters' first description of a bilioenteric reconstruction more than 100 years ago, major technical advances have

[*] Corresponding author: Professor and Chairman Department of Surgical Division, Chief of Hepatobiliary and Pancreatic Surgery, Department of Surgery, Instituto Nacional de Ciencias Médicas y Nutrición "Salvador Zubirán", Vasco de Quiroga 15, Colonia Sección XVI, Delegación Tlalpan, CP 14000, México City, México. Tel: +52 (55) 5487 0900, email: miguel.mercadod@quetzal.innsz.mx.

[†] Fellow of Hepatobiliary and Pancreatic Surgery, Instituto Nacional de Ciencias Médicas y Nutrición "Salvador Zubirán," email: drjulioalfaro@hotmail.com.

occurred through time. Bilioenteric anastomoses can be classified as extra-hepatic and intra-hepatic, depending of the anatomical area of the biliary tract used. Extra-hepatic anastomoses include choledo-choduodenostomy, choledochojejunostomy, and hepatojejunostomy. Intra-hepatic anastomoses include hepaticojejunostomy (Hepp-Couinaud) and peripheral cholangiojejunostomy (Longmire-Sanford). The Hepp-Couinaud technique is the most frequently performed anastomosis. This approach exposes the extra-hepatic course of the left hepatic duct and allows a wide anastomosis to a Roux-en-Y jejunal loop. The use of trans-anastomotic stents is no longer necessary and has limited indications. Complications of BEA include cholangitis, biliary fistula, intra-abdominal abscesses and strictures. Long-term follow-up report excellent results in 90% of the patients. Sixty-five percent of recurrent strictures develop during the first 2 years and 80% during the first 5- years after surgery. In this chapter we present the most frequently BEA techniques performed, their complications and outcome.

Introduction

Historical Background

Hepatobiliary diseases have been described in ancient manuscripts from civilizations dating centuries ago (Egypt, Greece, and Mesopotamia). [1] As knowledge of anatomy and physiology improved, breakthroughs occurred through time in the field of surgical treatment of hepatobiliary diseases. One of the first surgical interventions reported was surgical removal of gallstones by Fabricus in 1618. Jean-Louis Petit is considered as the founder of gall bladder surgery, suggesting the creation of biliary fistula in 1733. [1] Simms performed the first elective surgery for jaundice in 1878 (Cholecystostomy). Langenbuch iconic first cholecystectomy in 1882, opened a new era in hepatobiliary surgery. [2, 3] History of bilioenteric anastomoses (BEA) began with Winiwater (cholecystoenterostomy) in 1881, [4] Mayo (choledochoduodenostomy) in 1905, [4] followed by Monprofit's BEA (hepaticojejunostomy) using a Roux-en-Y intestinal loop. [4] Bilioenteric anastomoses continued to evolve with different modifications, as the mucosal graft technique described by Rodney-Smith and Hepp-Couinaud´s approach to intra-hepatic biliary tract. [4] Different techniques began to be used for challenging bilioenteric anastomoses, some of these techniques were described by Longmire-Sanford (partial liver resection) and Blumgart (hilar dissection for intra-hepatic anastomoses). [5] Gupta et al. [6] has even published the use of the appendix for hepaticoporto-appendico-jejunostomy for biliary atresia. [6] In 1986, Mouret performed the first laparoscopic cholecystectomy [7] and since then, laparoscopic approach has become more important in surgery every day and is now being applied in BEA. These innovations couldn´t have been possible without the contribution of great anatomists and courageous surgeons that have played a crucial role through history of medicine and especially in the surgical field. New developments in tissue engineer will modify in the near future reconstructions of the biliary tract. [8, 9] Along with advancements in surgery, auxiliary methods have contributed to improve results. Interventional radiology, endoscopic treatment and modern imaging techniques have also allowed marked improvements in BEA.

Indications of Bilioenteric Anastomoses

A wide range of diseases that affects the biliary tract may cause biliary obstruction, stressing the need of surgical procedures (bilioenteric anastomoses) to adequately drain bile from the liver. Bilioenteric anastomoses are necessary to relieve bile outflow obstruction secondary to benign or malignant disease of the biliary tree, as well as secondary to surgical procedures in which the biliary tract has been surgically removed and needs to be reconstructed. The main objective of these derivations is to drain bile from the liver into the gastrointestinal tract, therefore, preventing short and long term complications as repeated episodes of cholangitis, secondary biliary cirrhosis, portal hypertension and eventually death.

The main indication for a bilioenteric derivation is to relieve obstructive jaundice, whether secondary to a benign or malignant disease or as part of reconstruction due to surgical resection of the biliary tract. Table 1 shows the most frequent etiologies of obstructive jaundice.

Not all causes of obstructive jaundice require a BEA; many problems can be actually treated by endoscopic or interventional radiology techniques. The type of anastomosis depends on the etiology of the obstruction or the type of surgical resection/reconstruction of the biliary tract and will be discuss with further detail in the chapter.

Table 1. Etiology of Obstructive Jaundice

Benign Etiology
• Choledocholithiasis
• Mirizzi's Syndrome
• Primary Sclerosing Cholangitis
• Biliary Tuberculosis
• Parasites (Ascaris lumbricoides, Liver flukes)
• Pancreatitis
• Biliary Strictures (Trauma, Iatrogenic, Radiation)
• Congenital Strictures (Atresia, Congenital Cysts)
Malignant Etiology
• Cholangiocarcinoma (Klatskins' Tumor, Distal cholangiocarcinoma)
• Pancreatic Cancer
• Ampullary Carcinomas
• Gallbladder Cancer
• Secondary Adenopathies in the Porta Hepatis

Types of Anastomoses

Different types of BEA have been described along history. Many are considered obsolete and have only historical value. We classify BEA according to the anatomical location of the biliary tract that will be used and the gastrointestinal viscera that is going to be anastomosed to the biliary tract.

Bilioenteric Anastomoses can be classified into two types [10]:

1) Extrahepatic Anastomoses
   - Choledochoduodenostomy, Choledochojejunostomy
   - Cholecystojejunostomy, Cholescystoduodenostomy
   - Hepatojejunostomy
2) Intrahepatic Anastomoses
   - Central Cholangiojejunostomy
     a) Hepaticojejunosotomy (Hepp-Couinaud)
     b) Rodney-Smith (mucosal graft)
     c) Abdo-Machado

- Peripheral Cholangiojejunostomy
    a) Longmire-Sanford
    b) Dogliotti
    c) Soupault-Couinaud

Extrahepatic Anastomoses

Cholecystojejunostomy, Cholecystoduodenostomy and Chole-cystogastrostomy

The gallbladder can be anastomosed to different parts of the gastrointestinal tract, and that will determine the type of anastomosis. These procedures include anastomosis to the jejunum, stomach and duodenum. They have the advantage of being a technically easy procedure. Cholecystojejunostomy for palliation of jaundice in advanced pancreatic and periampullary cancer is safe and well established. [11] Anastomoses to the gallbladder should be avoided as far as possible, and it should only be reserved for palliation with proven distal carcinoma and if the patient is expected to live a few months. [12] The only contraindications are the involvement of the cystic duct by tumor or a low cystic duct insertion. [13] The junction of the cystic duct and the common hepatic duct has to be at least 1 cm away from the malignant obstruction. The disadvantage is that the gallbladder usually becomes infected and has a major risk of perforation and cholangitis. [12] The type of anastomoses does not appear to have much effect on the complication rate. [12] Roux-en-Y cholecystojejunostomy seems to improve the complication rates, but it has the disadvantage of being more ulcerogenic.[12] Hepatojejunostomy is preferred over these anastomoses, the more distant this surgical bypass is from the gallbladder duct, the less likely it is to be involved early in the progression of the disease. [14-18]

Laparoscopic approach is an option for this type of procedures. Laparoscopic cholecystojejunostomy is the most often performed palliative procedure being much easier than laparoscopic hepatojejunostomy, but has the disadvantage of the same negative results as the open technique. [18-19]

Choledochoduodenostomy

Anastomoses between the common bile duct and the duodenum may be performed end-to-end or side-to-side, being the former more frequently done. They are indicated in the treatment of multiple calculi of the common bile duct, retained stones, distal common bile duct strictures, ampullary stenosis, benign ampullary tumors, [20] dilated common bile duct (>20mm), failure of endoscopic retrograde cholangiopancreatography (ERCP) or not availability of ERCP.[21-25] It has the advantage that guarantees physiological bile flow into the duodenum and endoscopic anastomoses control. The main disadvantage of the procedure is ascending cholangitis and "sump syndrome". [23, 26-28]

Many authors now advocate laparoscopic choledochoduodenostomy as a safe and effective procedure. [29-31] Laparoscopic BEA have to be performed in highly specialized centers under trained personnel. Endoscopic ultrasonography-guided choledochoduodenostomy can be safely performed and is now being described by some groups. [32] Nevertheless, some authors consider Choledochoduodenostomy as an obsolete procedure. [33-35] Choledochoduodenostomy is contraindicated in common bile duct <15mm, perivaterian diverticulum and sclerosing cholangitis. [36]

Choledochojejunostomy

Choledochojejunostomy is the anastomoses between the common bile duct and a Roux-en-Y jejunal loop. The main indications are benign; mainly iatrogenic, biliary strictures and malignant obstruction of the biliary tract caused by pancreatic or duct wall tumors. [37] A defunctionalized intestinal loop of the proximal jejunum is used to construct a Roux-en-Y anastomosis to the biliary tract, preventing in this manner the reflux of food debris. Laparoscopic approach has also been proposed for this type of anastomoses. [38] The anastomoses can be performed side-to-side or end-to-side. Roux-en-Y anastomoses was established to reduce the "Sump syndrome"; nevertheless, it doesn´t completely eliminates the risk of postoperative cholangitis [39-41] and is associated with other serious complications unique to this procedure, such as jejunal loop herniation, intussusception, variceal jejunal loop hemorrhage [42, 43] and Roux-en-Y limb-associated motility abnormality that can also lead to enterobiliary reflux. [44] Contraindications for this procedure are patients with a short life expectancy (< 6 months) and with very poor functional status. [45] Patients not suited for this BEA should undergo less invasive palliative procedures, including percutaneous biliary drainage or endoscopic stenting.

Hepatojejunostomy

It consists of anastomoses between the common hepatic duct and a Roux-en-Y jejunal loop. It can be performed end-to-side or side-to-side. The main indications are benign strictures, generally iatrogenic bile duct injuries, [46] biliary fibrosis secondary to chronic pancreatitis and previous bilioenteric procedures that suffer stenosis. Among malignant indications are cholangiocarcinoma and gallbladder carcinoma that infiltrates the common bile duct, and is considered as a final step for palliative treatment. [47] End-to-side anastomoses are preferred over side-to-side, because the latter cannot eliminate the risk of tumor ingrowth and obliteration of the anastomoses. [37] Laparoscopic approach has also been proven to be a safe procedure. [48] The main contraindication for this technique is a short life expectancy (< 6 months).

Intrahepatic Anastomoses

Hepaticojejunostomy (Hepp-Couinaud)

This technique was first described in 1956 by Hepp and Couinaud as an approach to the extrahepatic course of the left hepatic bile duct. [49] This technique is also known as segment 3 hepatojejunostomy or B3 cholangiojejunostomy. [50] The most common indication are benign strictures, especially iatrogenic bile duct injuries. It is particularly useful in high strictures (benign or malignant) just below the confluence of the left and right hepatic duct. [51] Hepp-Couinaud approach in bile duct injury is the most frequent type of reconstruction technique performed. It has the advantage of allowing anastomoses over adequate tissue to ensure a high quality anastomoses. Contraindications for this procedure are the presence of an atrophic left lobe, a percentage of hepatic parenchyma to be drained less than 30% or less than two segments and presence of portal hypertension. [52-53] It is a BEA that provides the best outcome and follow-up results.

Cholangiojejunostomy (Longmire-Sanford)

It was described in 1949 by Longmire and Sanford as anastomoses to bile duct of segment II/III. This technique requires partial resection of segment III to expose dilated intrahepatic ducts and perform anastomoses to a Roux-en-Y jejunal loop. [55] The main indication for this procedure is proximal malignant obstruction of the biliary tract as a palliative treatment. The main complications of this technique are bleeding and dysfunction of the anastomoses. Less invasive maneuvers are preferred, such as percutaneous trans-hepatic biliary drainage. This type of procedure is now rarely performed due to better palliative procedures with less morbidity.

Techniques

The main objective of all BEA techniques is to accomplish adequate biliary outflow into the gastrointestinal tract. Several principles must be achieved to obtain a high quality anastomoses: [56]

- Tension free anastomoses
- Well vascularized
- Widely patent anastomoses
- Mucosa-to-Mucosa
- Anastomoses that drain all parts of the liver

In the present chapter we will discuss the most frequently performed bilioenteric anastomoses; the technical aspects of Roux-en-Y anastomosis will not be mentioned with detail.

Type of Suture

The types of sutures utilized are important for adequate functioning of the anastomoses. The ideal suture is hydrolysable monofilament absorbable 4-0 or 5-0. Multiple knots are avoided and should be placed outside the lumen to prevent sludge formation and bile stasis. Silk and Catgut are not recommended due to intense inflammatory response generated. Generally, anastomoses are monolayer with interrupted stitches, but a continuous suture can be used if the anastomosis is wide or according to the surgeon's preference.

Recommended sutures:

- Polyglicolic acid
- Polydioxanone
- Polypropylene monofilament
- Polyglecaprone 25

Cholecystojejunostomy (Open Technique)

Incisions

Different types of incisions may be used to explore the abdomen. A right subcostal incision with or without a vertical extension is an excellent option (Hockey stick). A bilateral subcostal incision (Chevron) can also be used or a midline incision. (Figure 1).

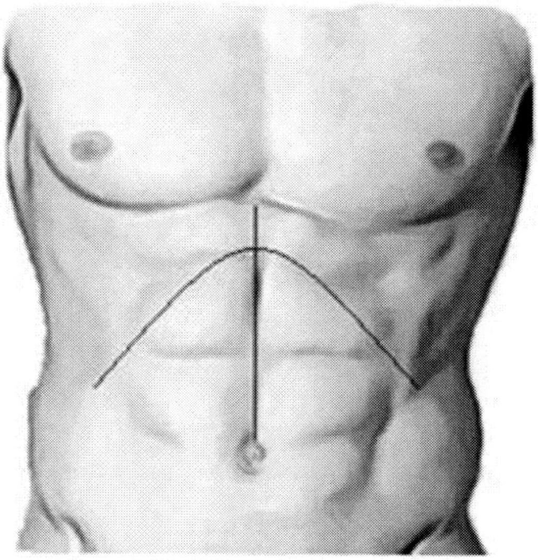

Figure 1. Types of incisions.

Surgical Aspects

Once the abdominal cavity has been reached, the surgeon must be sure that the cystic duct insertion is at least 1 cm away from the tumor and that the cystic duct is patent. The Gallbladder is left in situ and the body is used for the anastomosis. A simple jejunal loop that reaches the sub-hepatic space in an easy and tension free manner is used, or if the surgeon's preference is a Roux-en-Y jejunal limb is used and passed in a retrocolic or antecolic manner. The jejunum is approximated to the gallbladder using a posterior row of interrupted absorbable sutures (3-0). The body of the gallbladder is opened and the incision is prolonged as much as possible (at least 2-3 cm).

The anti-mesenteric border of the jejunum is opened in a parallel manner, but shorter. Full thickness of the gallbladder and jejunal wall is included in the anastomoses, using continuous absorbable sutures (3-0 or 4-0). The anastomoses begin in the middle (posterior wall) and runs to both corners; once the corner is reached, the anterior wall anastomoses is continued using Connell stitches. The anterior serosal layer is not necessary to approximate. A drain may be left in place. (Figure 2).

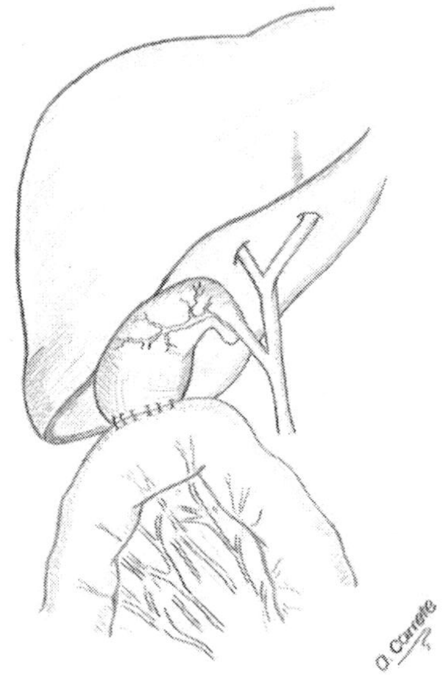

Figure 2. Anastomoses between the Gallbladder and a jejunal loop.

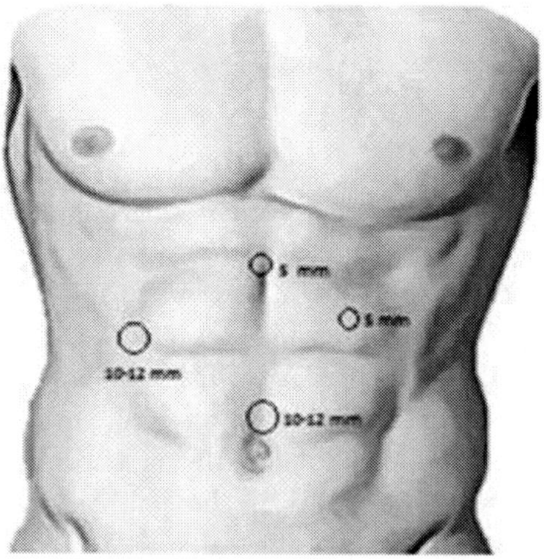

Figure 3. Laparoscopic port placement.

Cholecystojejunostomy (Laparoscopic)

Port Placement

The patient is placed in a supine position and the surgeon is placed in the right side or standing between the legs of the patient. Four ports are necessary. The first port is placed periumbilically (10-12 mm), a second (5 mm) subxiphoid trocar is placed, a third port (10-12 mm) placed in the right subcostal area in the nipple line and the fourth port (5 mm) is placed in the left upper quadrant. (Figure 3).

Surgical Aspects

A 30 degree-angle scope is recommended. Once the ports are placed, a general inspection of the abdominal cavity is performed and the organs to anastomose are evaluated. The jejunal loop to be used is verified that it reaches tension free and easily the sub-hepatic space. A cholecystostomy and jejunostomy is performed using cautery or ultrasonic scalpel. Two stay sutures can be placed to aid during the anastomoses. Side-to-side anastomosis is performed using an endoscopic stapler (45 mm length and 2.5 mm thickness). (Figure 4) The common enterotomy can be closed with interrupted absorbable suture (3-0) or using a second cartridge of stapler. A close drain is placed.

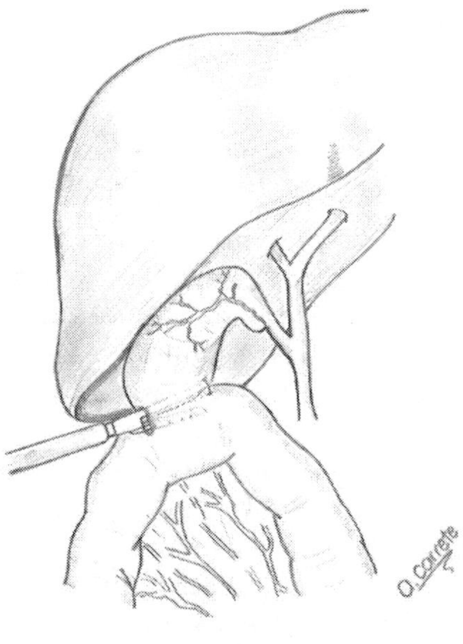

Figure 4. Laparoscopic cholecystojejunostomy using and endoscopic stapler.

Choledochoduodenostomy (Side-to-Side)

Incisions

A right subcostal incision with or without a vertical extension is an excellent option (Hockey stick). A bilateral subcostal incision (Chevron) can also be used or a midline incision. (Figure 5).

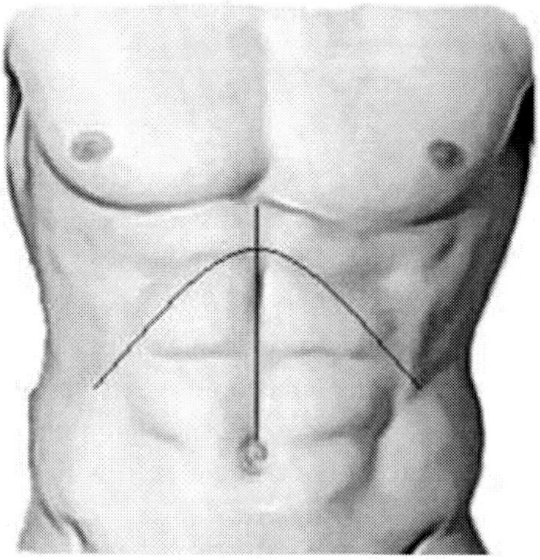

Figure 5. Types of incisions.

Surgical Aspects

The first step is to mobilize the colon inferiorly to allow adequate exposure of the gallbladder, duodenum and hepatoduodenal ligament. (Figure 6) If the patient has previous surgeries, careful dissection and adhesiolysis has to be performed. A Kocher maneuver is performed to allow adequate mobilization of the duodenum to the site of the planned anastomosis. Close attention must be paid to a tension free mobilization of the duodenum, being a critical step to achieve a tension free anastomosis. (Figure 7) Cholecystectomy is then performed in the classical manner. The hepatoduodenal ligament is incised and a dilated common bile duct is exposed. Stay sutures (3-0) are placed laterally to help with exposition and traction. Extensive dissection of the bile duct has to be avoided. A choledochotomy is performed of at least 2.5 cm, close to the proximal superior border of the duodenum. A perpendicular longitudinal duodenotomy is performed that has to be smaller than the choledochotomy. (Figure 8) The posterior wall anastomoses are performed using interrupted absorbable sutures (3-0 or 4-0) (Figure 9). The first suture is placed in the 6 o′clock position and more sutures are placed to the 3 o′clock and 9 o′clock position. The sutures must include all the wall of the common bile duct and duodenum. The sutures are tied and the stay sutures are released. All sutures are cut but the ones placed in the 3 o′clock and 9 o′clock position. The anterior wall anastomosis is performed with interrupted absorbable sutures (3-0 or 4-0) making sure the knot is left outside. Too many sutures are not recommended. A close drain is placed.

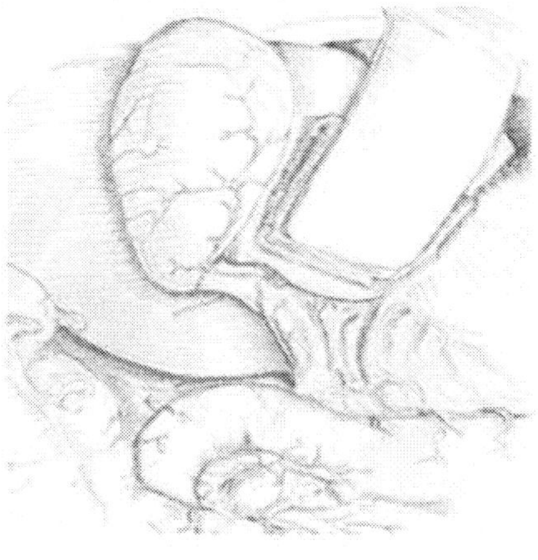

Figure 6. Adequate exposition of the gallbladder, duodenum and hepatoduodenal ligament is achieved after inferior mobilization of the colon.

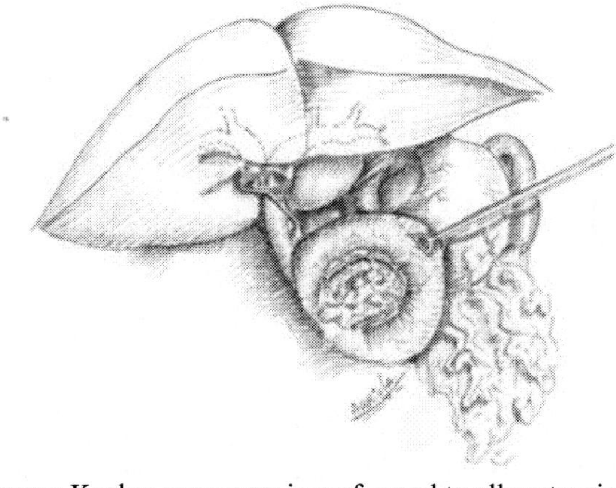

Figure 7. A generous Kocher maneuver is performed to allow tension-free anastomoses.

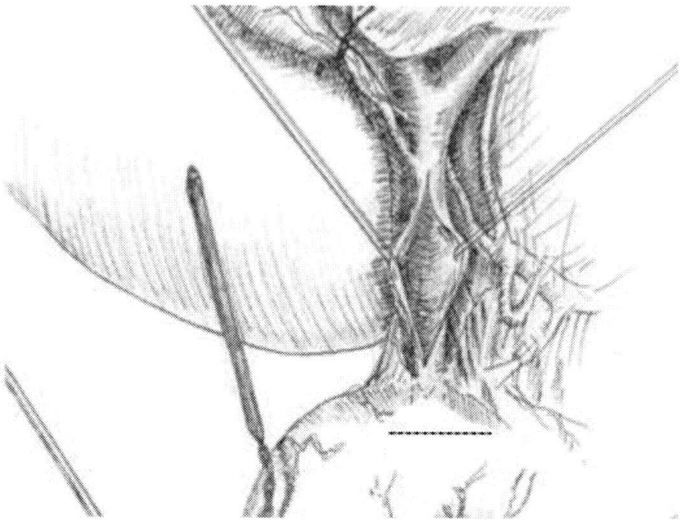

Figure 8. The common bile duct is exposed and stay sutures are placed to help with traction, a choledochotomy of at least 2.5 cm is performed close to the superior border of the duodenum that will be anastomosed and the enterotomy is performed perpendicular to the choledochotomy (solid line).

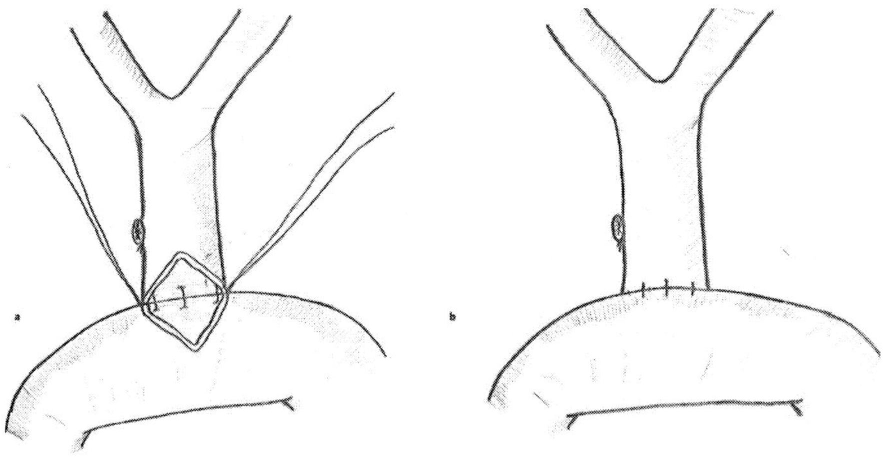

Figure 9. *(a)* Posterior wall anastomoses using interrupted sutures, stay sutures are placed to help with traction. *(b)* Final appearance of the Choledochoduodenostomy.

Choledochojejunostomy (Side-to-side)

Incisions

A right subcostal incision with or without a vertical extension is an excellent option (Hockey stick). A bilateral subcostal incision (Chevron) can also be used or a midline incision. Chevron incision provides the best exposure. (Figure 10).

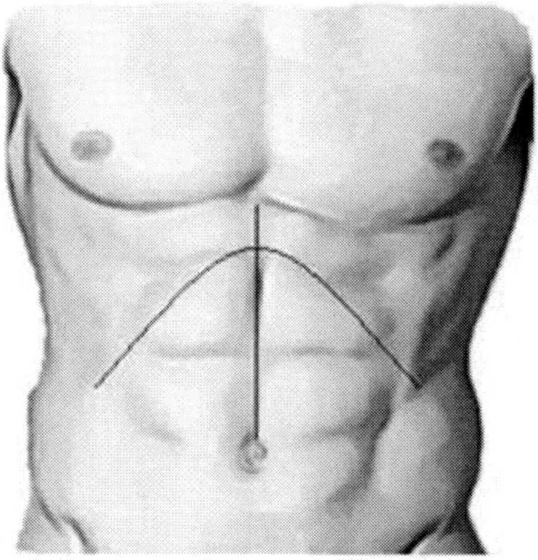

Figure 10. Types of incisions.

Surgical Aspects

The colon must be mobilized inferiorly to allow adequate exposure of the hepatoduodenal ligament. In redo operations adhesiolysis must be carefully done. Cholecystectomy is performed in the traditional manner. Once the cystic duct has been ligated it can be used as a reference landmark to be followed to its junction with the common bile duct; the hepatic artery can also be used as a reference landmark. A fine-needle syringe can be of aid in the identification of the biliary tract or intraoperative ultrasound can also be used. As the hepatoduodenal ligament has been opened and the common bile duct identify, care must be taken to avoid excessive dissection of the biliary tract to avoid injury to axial vascular structures. Sutures (3-0 or 4-0) that serve as traction are placed laterally and above the area of stricture. A Roux-en-Y jejunal limb is prepared for the anastomosis. The common bile duct is opened (at least 2 cm) and is cleared of stones and sludge using randall forceps and biliary fogartys. A smaller enterotomy is performed in the antimesenteric border of the jejunal limb at 5 cm from the close end using cautery or ultrasonic scalpel. The anastomosis is started with sutures on both corners, and interrupted absorbable sutures (4-0) are placed with 3mm distance and include all the wall of the common bile duct and jejunum. (Figure 11) The anterior wall anastomosis is performed in the same manner. A close drain is placed. (Figure 12).

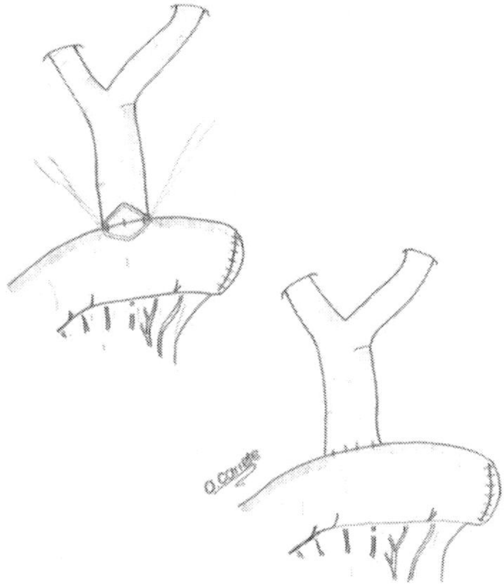

Figure 11. Choledochojejunostomy with a Roux-en-Y jejunal loop.

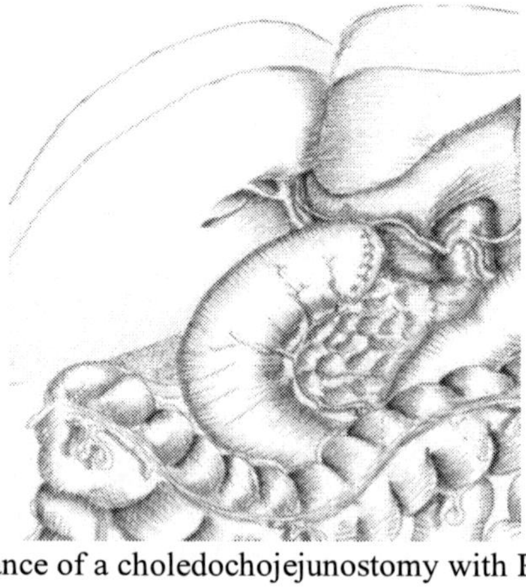

Figure 12. Final appearance of a choledochojejunostomy with Roux-en-Y retrocolic jejunal limb.

Hepatojejunostomy (End-to-Side)

Incisions

A right subcostal incision with or without a vertical extension is an excellent option (Hockey stick). A bilateral subcostal incision (Chevron) can also be used or a midline incision. Chevron incision provides the best exposure (Figure 13).

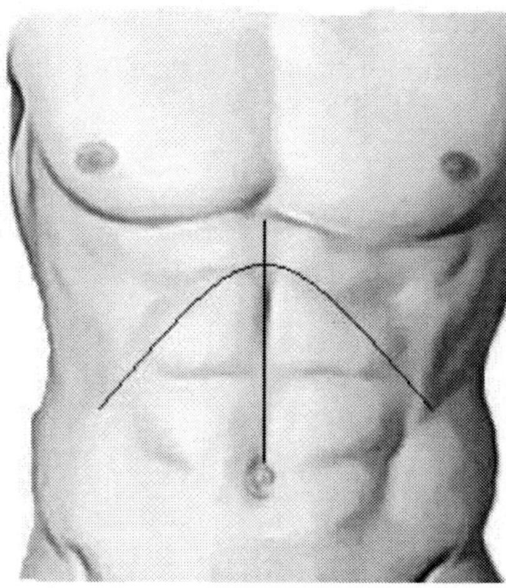

Figure 13. Types of incisions.

Surgical Aspects

Once the abdominal cavity has been reached, adequate mobilization of structures is of great importance. The colon is mobilized inferiorly and the hepatoduodenal ligament is adequately exposed. The common hepatic duct is searched by opening the heptoduodenal ligament. A fine needle-syringe may be used to find the bile duct. Once the bile duct has been exposed, stay sutures (3-0) that aid in traction are placed laterally above the area of stricture. The common bile duct is ligated below the area of stricture and transected between the ligatures. After adequately exposing the common hepatic duct, a Roux-en-Y jejunal loop is position in a retrocolic manner into the subhepatic space (Figure 14a). Excessive dissection has to be avoided of the proximal stump. The proximal biliary tract is cleaned from stones and sludge with saline irrigation and the use of randall forceps or biliary fogartys. An enterotomy is performed in the antimesenteric border of the jejunal limb at 5 cm from the close end. A suture can be placed in the anterior wall of the hepatic duct to be used as traction. It is important to create mucosa-to-mucosa anastomoses. The posterior wall anastomoses is performed from left to right using interrupted absorbable sutures (4-0 or 5-0) that are placed first in the posterior wall of the common hepatic duct in an outside/inside manner and into the jejunal limb Inside/outside. It has to be noticed that these are tied until the last suture is placed; keeping each suture in an orderly fashion to avoid crossing of the sutures. The knots are left outside the lumen. After the posterior wall anastomoses is performed, the anterior wall anastomoses is performed with interrupted absorbable sutures (4-0 or 5-0). A close drain is placed (Figure 14b).

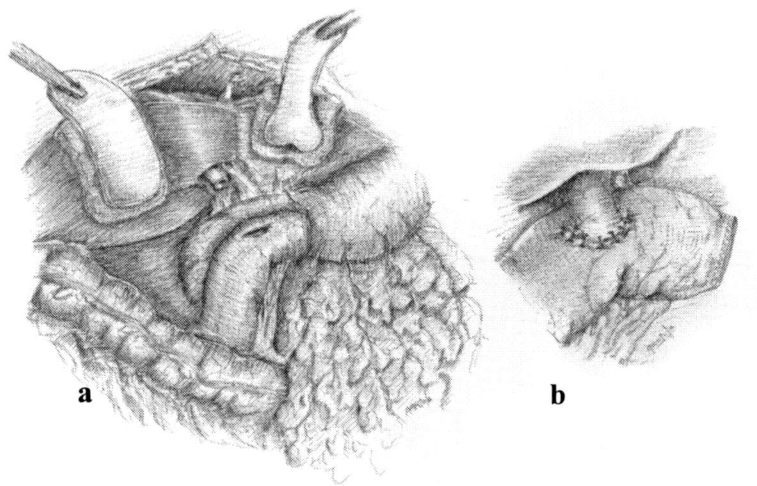

Figure 14. (a) The common hepatic duct is exposed and the Roux-en-Y jejunal limb is placed in the sub-hepatic space. (b) Final appearance of the hepatojejunostomy.

Hepaticojejunostomy (Hepp-Couinaud)

Incisions

A right subcostal incision with or without a vertical extension is an excellent option (Hockey stick). A bilateral subcostal incision (Chevron) can also be used or a midline incision. Chevron incision provides the best exposure. The authors preferred approach is a right subcostal incision. (Figure 15)

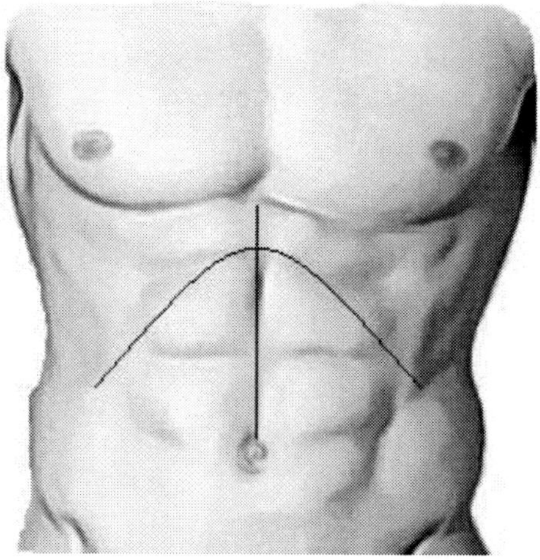

Figure 15. Types of incisions.

Surgical Aspects

Patients that undergo this procedure usually have previous surgeries. If it's a redo surgery careful dissection has to be done and the small intestine has to be revised for any previous Roux-en-Y anastomoses. The hilar plate is carefully dissected. To achieve adequate exposure of the left duct, the hepatoduodenal ligament is opened at hilar plate level. (Figure 16) Several maneuvers can be used to expose the left duct. Partial resection of segment IVb or V may be necessary to lower the hilar plate. (Figure 17) This can be safely performed and bleeding is easily controlled with cautery. The Champeau maneuver helps prolong the incision over the left bile duct, and consists of transection of liver bridge between liver segment IVb and left lateral segments. Once the extrahepatic course of the left hepatic duct is exposed, an incision over the anterior surface of the left duct is performed. (Figure 18) Minor bleeding can be controlled with hemostatic sutures of monofilament (5-0). The biliary tract is cleaned with saline irrigation and dilators are introduced to confirm the anatomy of the ducts. A Roux-en-Y jejunal loop is performed and brought up to the hepatic hilum in a retrocolic manner. Stay sutures are placed in the anterior border of the open duct to help exposure (Figure 19). Enterotomy is performed in the antimesenteric border of the jejunal limb at approximately 5 cm from the close end. Side-to-side (mucosa-to-mucosa) anastomoses is performed with interrupted absorbable sutures (4-0 or 5-0); placed outside/inside through the bile duct and inside/outside in the jejunum. (Figure 20) The sutures are placed from left to right and are not tied until the last suture of the posterior wall has been placed. After the posterior wall anastomoses is finished, the anterior wall is performed in the same manner with interrupted absorbable sutures (4-0 or 5-0). The jejunal limb is fixed to the liver capsule and a close drain is placed. (Figure 21).

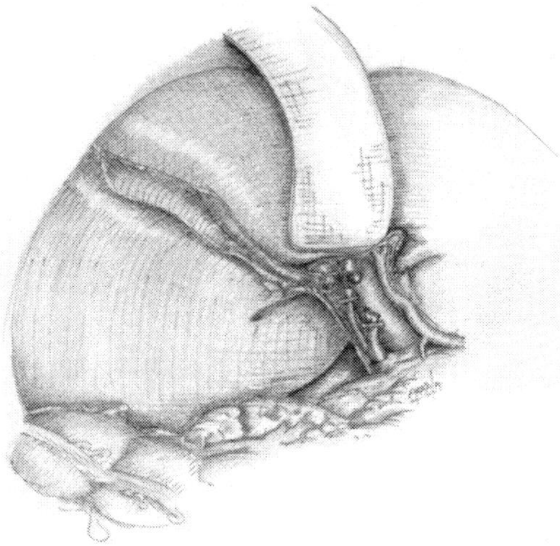

Figure 16. The hilar plate is dissected to expose the biliary tract confluence.

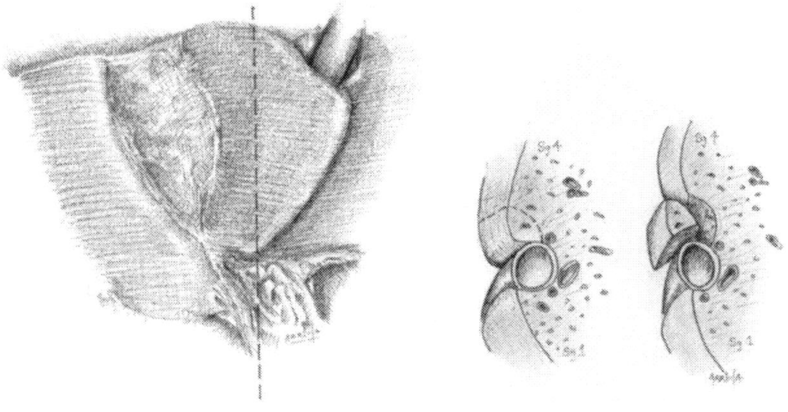

Figure 17. Partial resection of segment IV-V is performed to lower the hilar plate and expose the extrahepatic course of the left hepatic duct. The incision is done parallel to the hilar plate, between the gallbladder fossa and the round ligament. The dotted line is the limit between segment IV and V.

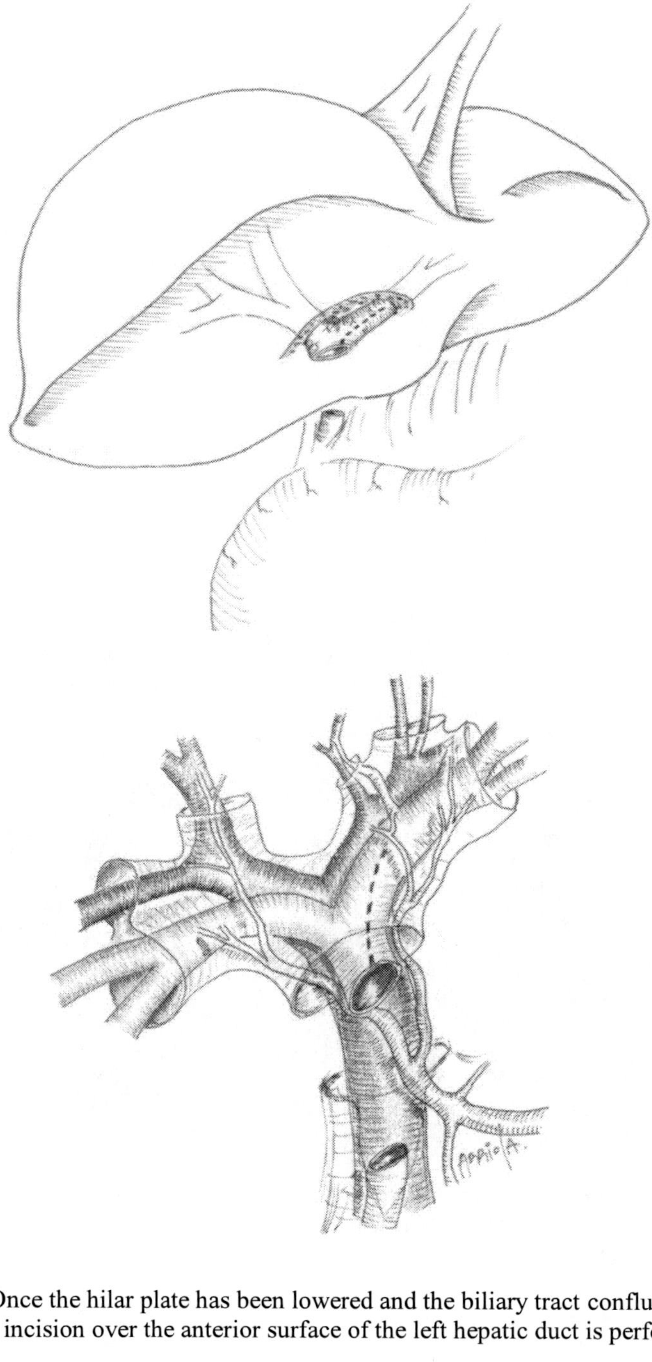

Figure 18. Once the hilar plate has been lowered and the biliary tract confluence exposed, an incision over the anterior surface of the left hepatic duct is performed.

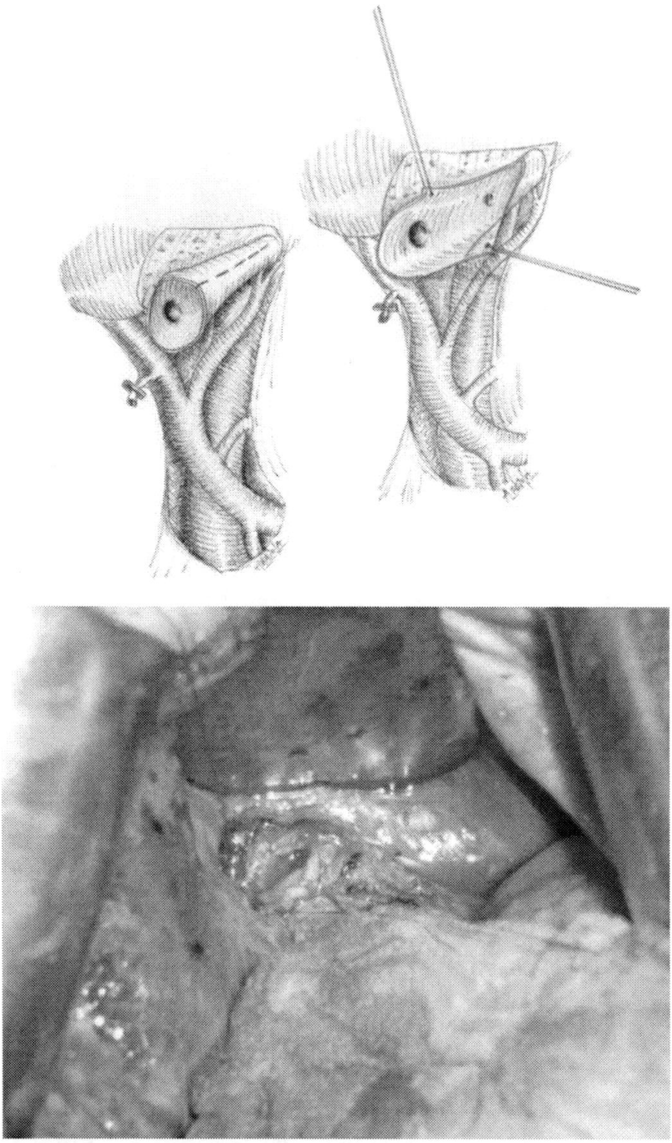

Figure 19. After the extrahepatic course of the left duct is opened, stay sutures are placed to help exposition of the biliary tract lumen, and dilators are introduce to identify the anatomy.

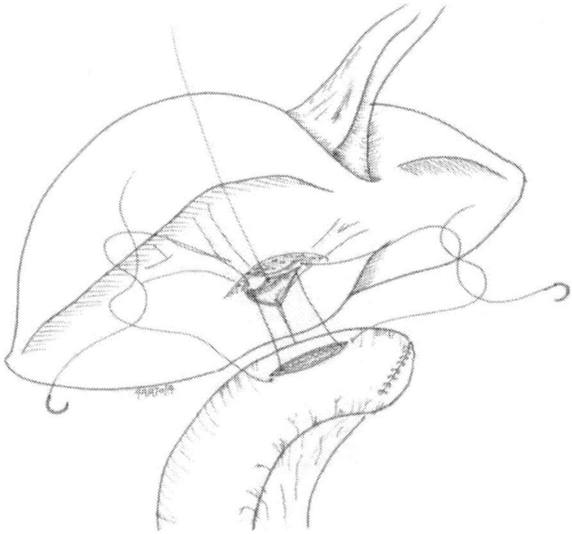

Figure 20. Absorbable hydrolysable monofilament sutures (5-0) are placed on both corners, outside/inside in the biliary tract and inside/outside in the jejunal loop.

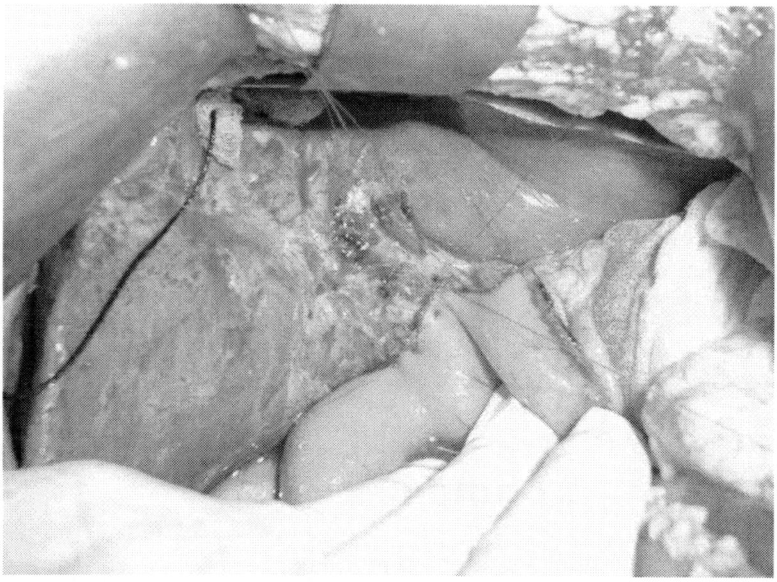

Figure 21. Final view of the Hepp-Couinaud anastomosis with intestinal loop fixed to the liver capsule.

To Stent Or Not to Stent a Bilioenteric Anastomoses?

Controversy exists with regards the use of stents or not in bilioenteric anastomoses. The author doesn´t uses stents in a routinely manner.

Benefits of stents:

- Preventing dehiscence by control of ductal and jejunal limb pressure.
- Prevents stenosis.
- Allows manipulation and/or dilation of the anastomoses in the postoperative period.
- Allows radiological control of the anastomoses.

Disadvantages of stents:

- No data supporting its routine use.
- Duration of stent placement is random and depends on the surgeon´s experience.
- Use of stents is cause of complications.
- They cause inflammatory reaction and cause bile stasis.

When bilioenteric anastomoses are performed electively, without cholangitis or infection, with a normal biliary tract (not dilated); stents are not necessary. Mercado et al. [57] reported more postoperative complications in patients with stents, including neo-formation of bile stones and complex fistulas (arterio-biliary and bilio-pleural fistulas). There is no benefit demonstrated with the use of biliary acids to prevent stent occlusion. [58]

The author recommends the use of stent in the following situations:

1) Thin bile ducts with diameter less than 4 mm.
2) Inflammation of the anastomosed ducts.

Complications

Bilioenteric anastomoses represent major surgical procedures and postoperative complications are divided into early and late complications. Many patients are acutely or chronically ill, making them more susceptible to suffer postoperative complications. Complications after BEA may require reoperation and result in long-term morbidity. [59] Early postoperative morbidity rate for BEA is 20-30% and mortality rate 0-2%. [60-63]

The most frequent early postoperative complication following BEA is wound infection (8-12%). [62, 63] Other early complications are cholangitis (5.7%), biloma/ intra-abdominal abscess (3.4%), biliary fistula, biliary-enteric anastomosis dehiscence, peritonitis and death (0-2%). [62, 64, 65] There are several factors associated to complications, such as patient's age, co-morbid conditions, and type of anastomosis performed, influencing outcome of BEA. [59] Other factors that should be considered as risk factors for complications are bile duct injuries, specifically when associated to vasculobiliary injuries.

Some postoperative complications have worst outcome and can potentially lead to reoperation, prolong hospital stay and death. Bile leakage is one of the major postoperative complications because is an important cause of morbidity and extended hospital stays. [66] Bile leakage secondary to BEA is presents in 4.6% of the cases. [62] The placement of drains helps detect this complication in the early postoperative period, allowing different treatments to prevent major complications.

Bile leakage is defined as [67]:

a) Bile discharge from an abdominal wound and/or drain, with a total bilirubin level of >5mg/mL or three times the serum level.
b) Intra-abdominal collections of bile confirmed by percutaneous aspiration.
c) Cholangiographic evidence of dye leaking from the opacified bile ducts.

Bile leaks can also be classified as minor and major. Minor bile leaks are small, manifested as self-limited drainage of bile-containing fluid via an external drain or as small postoperative sub-hepatic collections which resolve spontaneously. Major bile leaks include biliary fistulas, bilomas, bile ascites or bile peritonitis. [68] Bile drainage of more than 100 cc per day over a period of 2 weeks is unlikely to close spontaneously without manifesting long-term complications. [68]

Many patients don´t develop a clear fistula, but show a biloma; which is a confined collection of bile, usually in juxtaposition to the source of a bile leak. [68] Imaging techniques as abdominal ultrasound and Computer Tomography (CT) will show a large low density collection, its location and morphology. [69] Bilomas can be treated by interventional radiology by percutaneous drainage. Imaging is usually not indicated unless there is suspicion of early or late complications developing, and the most important evaluation tool is daily clinical assessment.

Late complications of BEA are strictures of the anastomoses. Several imaging techniques are available to confirm patency or stricture of the anastomosis. Radiological evaluation of the anastomosis should be performed whenever strictures are suspected. Magnetic Resonance Cholangio-pancreatography (MRCP) has proved to be a reliable noninvasive technique to visualize the biliary anastomosis. [70] The disadvantage of MRCP is that it is not easily available in many hospitals.

Katz et al. [71] described that sensitivity and specificity of MRCP was of 94.4% and 88.9%, respectively, with positive and negative predictive values of 94.4% and 89.9%, respectively. Beltrán et al. [72] had a sensitivity of 93%, and specificity of 97.6%, with a global diagnostic accuracy of 95.6%. MRCP is an excellent non-invasive method to evaluate BEA.

Once strictures are confirmed, Endoscopic Retrograde Cholangio-pancreatography (ERCP) or Percutaneous Transhepatic Cholangiography is used as a therapeutic instrument. Cantwell et al. [73] analyzed the effectiveness of percutaneous balloon dilation (PBBD) (Figure 22) as treatment of benign postoperative biliary strictures and the probability of a patient not having clinically significant restenosis at 2.5 and 3 years after primary PBBD was 0.66 and 0.56, respectively. Previous studies demonstrated that 38%–67% of patients did not have clinically significant stenosis. [74-76].

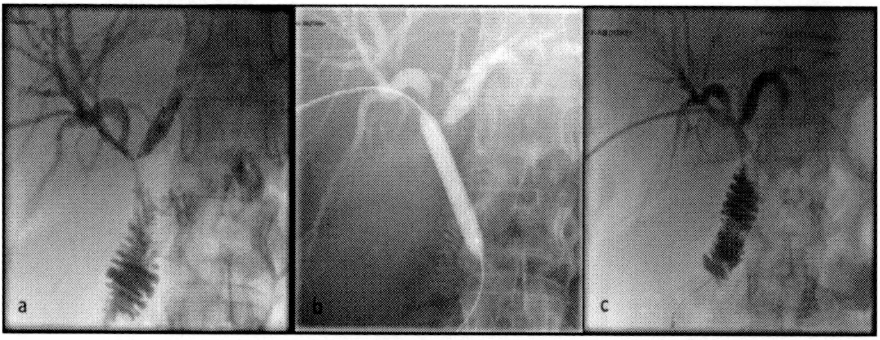

Figure 22. *(a)* Stenosis of the BEA is evident through a percutaneous trans-hepatic cholangiography. *(b)* Balloon dilation is being performed by interventional radiology. *(c)* Control cholangiography demonstrates the patency of the BEA after balloon dilation.

Cholecystojejunostomy

Many long-term complications will not be observed in different BEA, because they are performed in patients with malignant disease. Oishi et al. [77] reported a morbidity of 32% and late complications in 15% of the cases, including recurrent biliary stones with obstruction and anastomotic stricture; however, despite the morbidity, 85% of patients had a successful and durable biliary decompression during an 8 year follow-up. Cholecystojejunostomy is not the ideal BEA for benign disease, and it should be limited to malignant obstruction. Thomson et al. [78] described a series of patients in which all developed cholangitis and concluded that cholelithiasis and cholangitis are inevitable when this BEA is used for benign obstruction

Rare complications can occur and have been described as intussusception (cause of recurrent obstructive jaundice), right upper quadrant pain, cholangitis, or GI bleeding in patient with this BEA. [79] Bleeding varicose have been reported as late complications of palliative biliary surgery for chronic pancreatitis. [80, 81] Salam et al. [82] reported varices through the cholecystojejunostomy in a patient with concomitant obstruction of the common bile duct and the portal vein.

Cholecystojejunostomy is not recommended for definitive treatment of benign disease. When a benign biliary obstruction is suspected, other BEA has to be considered, due to the survival of these patients and the risk of cholangitis and malignancy. [77, 78, 83] Gallbladder carcinoma is a possible late complication of cholecystojejunostomy and should be remembered when dealing with patients that had this BEA. [83] Cholecystojejunostomy has a risk of malignancy and is another important reason why this procedure is abandoned in benign obstruction.

Choledochoduodenostomy (CDD)

Choledochoduodenostomy (CDD) is one of the BEA that has been more thoroughly described. Riedel was the first to describe them more than a century ago (1892). CDD is a controversial procedure; with a lot of complications described in the literature. Ascending cholangitis, sump syndrome and alkaline reflux gastritis are some of the documented complications. Although it has good long-term results in some studies, it is not the best procedure for lower common bile duct obstruction. [84] The most common complications are intra-abdominal abscess (26%), wound infection (20%), and biliary leakage (13%). [44]

CDD has a morbidity of 23% and a mortality of 3%. [86] CDD risk for cholangitis is between 0% to 12%, usually associated with stricture of the anastomosis and remnant or recurrent stones. [86] The width of CDD anastomoses has been of debate for some time, considered by some authors to range between 2-2.5 cm. Stricture of the anastomoses and subsequent development of cholangitis are the most frequently described long-term complications, and to avoid it several authors recommend a BEA width of at least 2. 0 cm. Several authors recommend a stoma size greater than 2.5 cm to prevent cholangitis. [87]

Sphincter of Oddi regulates the flow of bile and pancreatic juice into the duodenum preventing reflux of duodenal content back into the biliary tract, function that is lost with CDD. CDD is associated to pneumobilia, regurgitation of food debris and duodenal content into the biliary tract. [88] Although CDD are one of the most physiological BEA allowing bile outflow into the duodenum, most of its complications are associated to the loss of sphincter of Oddi function.

Side-to-side CDD has great risk of developing "sump syndrome." Sump syndrome is defined as the accumulation of biliary and duodenal contents in a poorly drained distal stump of the biliary tree. [89] Sump syndrome has been reported in 0 to 9.6% of the cases. [23, 90, 91] The presence of symptoms following food accumulation within the bile duct is what characterizes the syndrome. [92] Complications of sump syndrome are cholangitis, pancreatitis, hepatic abscesses, and secondary biliary cirrhosis. [92] Sump syndrome has a low incidence and appears to be related to BEA stricture and not a true sump syndrome. [89] Limiting the definition of sump syndrome to cholangitis and hepatic abscess may underreport true incidence of this syndrome. [44] (Figure 23).

Treatment of sump syndrome begins with endoscopic sphincterotomy in order to decompress the common bile duct, with good results. [93-96] Sometimes endoscopic treatment fails due to previous heavy or multiple stones, large food debris accumulated through the stoma that cannot be cleared with endoscopy. [92] Caroli-Bosc et al. [93] described their experience with patients with sump syndrome managed endoscopically and found out that 60% had food debris and 33% biliary calculi. Surgical treatment includes Roux-en-Y hepaticojejunostomy, with resection of the distal portion of the CBD. [92]

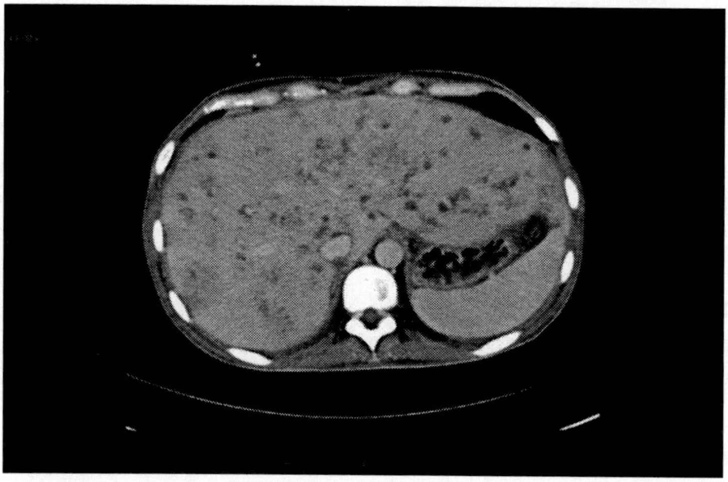

Figure 23. CT scan with multiple pericholangitic abscesses and mild dilation of intrahepatic bile ducts, suggestive of BEA stricture and ascending cholangitis.

The incidence of duodenogastric reflux (DGR) after CDD, assessed by endoscopy and histology, ranges from 11.5% to 70%, even though dyspeptic symptoms attributable to DGR have been reported in only 15% of patients. The symptoms related to DGR depend not only the presence but also in the severity of reflux; the presence of an intact pylorus in these patients could prevent the severity of DGR. [93] Lujan-Mompean et al. evaluated DGR in patients with cholecystectomy alone and in patients with cholecystectomy plus CDD. This last group had higher reflux rates than patients who underwent simple cholecystectomy, attributing it to unregulated bile flow to the duodenum following bypass of the sphincter of Oddi and altered motility of the pyloroduodenum due to surgical manipulation of the duodenum. [94] Most of the patients with CDD are asymptomatic and the degree of DGR does not necessarily produce symptoms in all patients. [93]

CDD have been associated to malignant. Reflux of food debris and substances into the biliary tract cause changes in the biliary epithelium that may lead to malignant transformation. [64] Eleftheriadis et al. [98] evaluated duct mucosa in patients who had a CDD performed and found that the mucosa showed hyperplasia, metaplastic goblet cells, and pyloric like gland formation; changes that are also found in patients with hepatolithiasis and congenital choledochal cyst, which have been considered as premalignant disease. [99, 100] Tocchi et al. [63] described an incidence of cholangiocarcinoma of 5.5% which was higher in patients with CDD, compared with hepaticojejunostomy or transduodenal sphincteroplasty (7.6% vs. 1.9% vs. 4.8%, respectively). Patients that underwent this type of BEA are recommended to have close follow-up in the long-term, especially if they had several episodes of cholangitis.

Choledochojejunostomy (CJ)

Most surgeons prefer a Roux-en-Y CJ in the management of benign biliary disease. [85] Postoperative morbidity of CJ is of 20% to 33%, with a mortality of 0% to 2%. [74, 100, 101] CJ are more complicated and takes longer; requiring circumferential dissection of the common bile duct and a Roux-en-Y anastomoses. [44] Hepaticojejunostomy is preferred over this BEA.

Hepaticojejunostomy

Hepaticojejunostomy has a morbidity rate of 19-49% and a mortality of 0-6% for benign disease [59, 100, 102-103] The most common complications include wound infection, cholangitis, bile leak, hemorrhage, pancreatitis, delayed gastric emptying, cardiopulmonary complications, systemic sepsis, renal failure, abscess formation, fistula formation, and stenosis. Factors associated to BEA complications are low serum albumin levels and worse American Association of Anesthesiologists (ASA) physical status. [59] Excellent results are expected in 90% of the cases when they are performed under expert hands.

Stricture following HJ occurs in 5% to 17%. [100, 102-104] Factors associated to stricture formation are vasculobiliary injuries, multiple repair attempts, biloma, external or internal biliary fistula, anastomosis in non-dilated duct, injury at or above the level of the biliary bifurcation, preoperative and postoperative percutaneous biliary drainage, and patient comorbidities. [74, 102] BEA strictures can be treated with endoscopic dilation, percutaneous dilation or redo surgery. Kucukay et al. [105] described the efficacy of percutaneous biliary balloon dilation (PBBD) of benign HJ strictures, and found a morbidity of 5.6%. Recurrent biliary stricture presents in two thirds of patients within 2–3 years after reconstruction, 80% of patients within 5 years, and 90% of patients within 7 years. [60, 106-107] Biliary leakage has been reported in 2.3% of the cases. [108] Initial management of biliary leakage may be with endoscopic treatment, interventional radiology and surgery in more complex cases. (Figure 24).

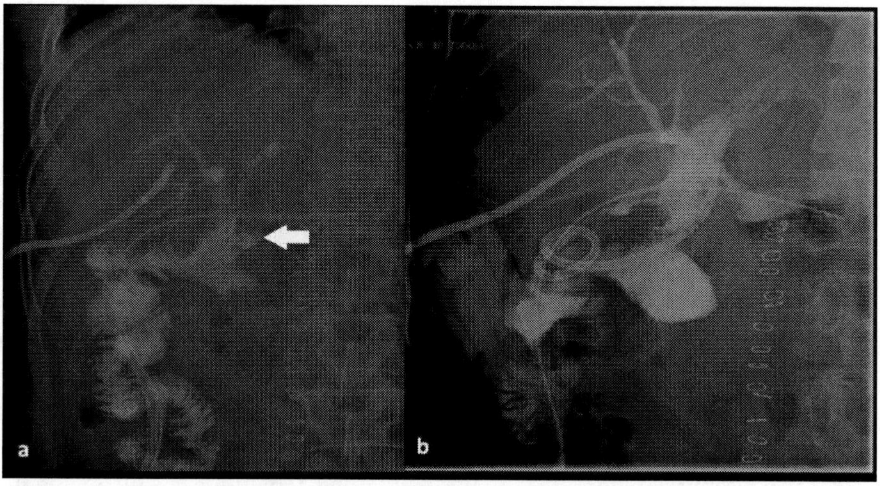

Figure 24. Image (*a*) corresponds to a percutaneous cholangiography through a previously placed external drainage catheter in which a biliary leakage (arrow) from the BEA was evident. Image (*b*) shows a percutaneous transhepatic internal-external catheter placed through the BEA to control the biliary fistula.

Outcome and Follow-Up

Time Interval and Duration of Follow-up

Time interval for follow-up after a bilioenteric anastomoses is of 3 months during the first year, every 6 months during the second year and yearly evaluation is recommended after the third year. The total minimum time interval for follow-up is of 5 years; when most bilioenteric anastomoses tend to dysfunction. Some author recommend follow-up for 2 to 5 years and other groups up to 10 to 20 years. [54, 60, 64, 109-110] It is important to remember that most patients with malignancy are not expected to reach this minimum time interval.

Laboratory Tests and Imaging

Several biochemical parameters and imaging techniques are used during follow-up to evaluate anastomoses patency:

- Liver function tests: Liver function test elevation after bilioenteric anastomoses is no infrequent. AST/ALT are highly sensible biomarkers of liver damage. Bilirrubin level is closely related to biliary obstruction. Alkaline phosphatase (AP) increase before there is clinical evidence of jaundice. In most cases AP levels return to normal value after bilioenteric anastomoses. AP persists high but with normal bilirubin levels when there is partial obstruction of a liver segment. [111] When total bilirubin and direct bilirubin levels rise, complete obstruction has to be ruled out. Many patients that undergo bilioenteric anastomoses never return to normal levels of AP and don't represent higher risk of cholangitis in the long-term.
- Liver Ultrasound (US): It is an imagine technique easily available. The disadvantage of this method is its limitation to evaluate liver hilum due to abundant interposition of structures and gas. It is useful to detect early complications as fluid collections. During follow-up it may evidence dilated intrahepatic bile ducts as a sign of BEA dysfunction.
- Computer Tomography (CT): It is useful in the diagnosis of early and late complications during the postoperative period and during follow-up.
- Magnetic Cholangioresonance: Is an excellent non-invasive method to evaluate patency of the anastomoses and is the first option for evaluating BEA. It has the disadvantage of not allowing any therapeutic action in the presence of obstruction. (Figure 25).
- Percutaneous cholangiography: It is used when cholangioresonance is not available. It has the advantage of allowing direct manipulation of the BEA if it is required with balloon dilation or drainage catheter need to be placed to control biliary leakage or progressive dilation of the BEA. (Figure 26)

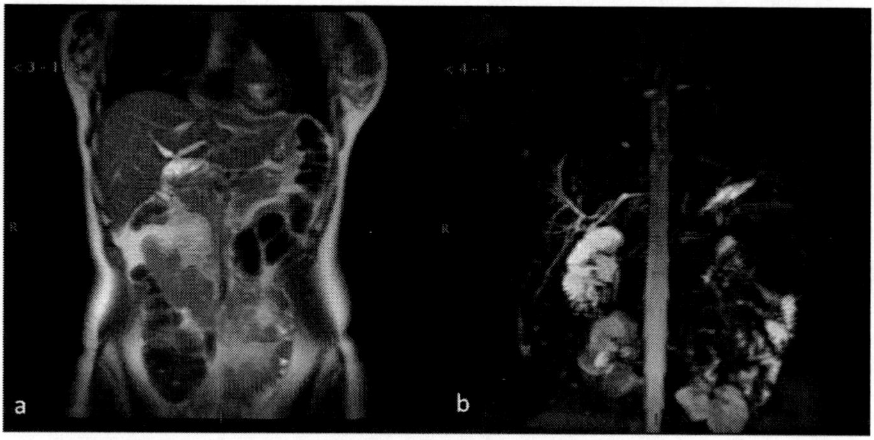

Figure 25. Image *(a)* corresponds to a T2 coronal magnetic cholangioresonance with a patent BEA. Image *(b)* corresponds to a 3D cholangioresonance volumetric reconstruction of a patent BEA with adequate biliary outflow into the jejunal limb in which the biliary tract has normal diameter.

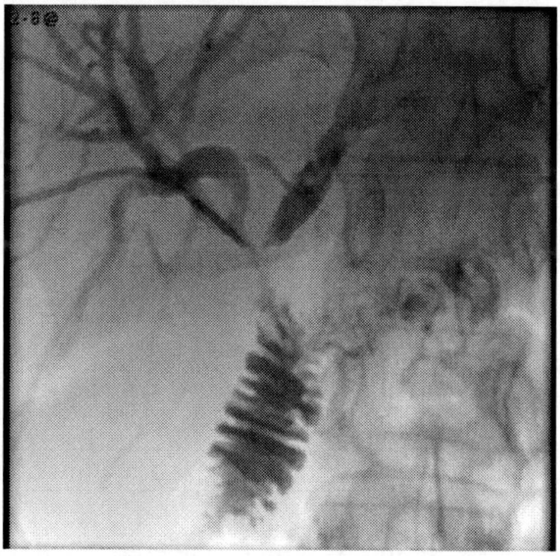

Figure 26. Percutaneous trans-hepatic cholangiography in which a stenotic BEA and dilation of the intrahepatic biliary tract is evident.

Imaging studies are not routinely indicated unless suspicion of early or late complications exists or stricture of the anastomoses needs to be ruled out during follow-up. Imaging studies are determined according to biochemical and clinical symptoms. Biochemical parameters are useful and are evaluated in every check-up.

Classifications

There are several classifications used to evaluate outcome and patency of bilioenteric anastomoses. These classifications include laboratory findings and clinical parameters. The most frequently used classifications are the Terblanche [110] scale (Table 2) and Mc Donald [65] classification. (Table 3).

Table 2. Terblanche Classification

Grade I	Excellent Results	No biliary symptoms with normal liver function test.
Grade II	Good Results	Transitory symptoms, currently no symptoms and normal liver function test.
Grade III	Fair Results	Clearly related symptoms requiring medical therapy and/or deteriorating liver function tests.
Grade IV	Poor Results	Recurrent stricture requiring correction or related death.

Table 3. McDonald Classification

Grade A	No clinical symptoms from the biliary tract, normal laboratory liver function tests.
Grade B	No clinical signs, laboratory liver function tests slightly elevated liver or periodical episodes of pain or fever.
Grade C	Pain, cholangitis with the presence of fever, jaundice and abnormal laboratory tests.
Grade D	Condition requiring surgical or endoscopic correction.

Patients with Grade A and B are considered as having an excellent outcome. These patients are amenable to follow-up twice a year to determine their clinical symptoms and laboratory findings. [65] In the case patients evolve to Grade C, the presence of cholangitis must be assessed, patency of the anastomosis and liver parenchyma status through US or cholangioresonance. The need for hospital stay and endoscopic, radiological or surgical treatment has to be evaluated. Grade C and D are considered as poor outcome; therefor, closer follow-up is recommended in this group. Follow-up is mandatory in all patients that undergo bilioenteric anastomoses because

60% of therapeutic failure occurred in the first 3 years and 80% during the first 5 years. [106, 107]

Three scenarios may occur in patients with Grade III or Grade C:

1) Recurrent episodes of cholangitis, abnormal liver function tests, normal liver parenchyma and a patent anastomosis. These cases are treated with antibiotics and ursodesoxycolic acid.
2) Episodes of cholangitis, abnormal liver function tests, especially AP, dilated intrahepatic bile ducts and stricture of the anastomosis. Treatment of choice is ERCP and/or interventional radiology and as last resource redo surgery.
3) Recurrent episodes of cholangitis, pericholangitic abscesses and stricture of the anastomosis. Treatment may begin with antibiotics, ERCP and/or interventional radiology, redo surgery with possible hepatectomy if less invasive strategies fail.

Good long-term results can be achieved in 70-90% of the cases. [112] The John Hopkins group reported a series of 142 patients with a success rate of 90.8% at 5 year follow-up [64] Other authors report successful results between 80-90% of the cases at 5 year follow-up. [113] The authors experience with 355 patients reported success in 94% of the cases (most of them secondary to iatrogenic bile duct injury). An important factor associated to successful results is the experience of the surgeon and patients that require complex biliary surgery and reconstruction should be referred to a specialized center.

Two-third of strictures will appear during the first 2 years and 90% during the first 5 years. [106] The authors recommendation for treatment of recurrent strictures is to begin with less invasive measures to dilate the anastomoses. When strictures occur, endoscocopic or transhepatic balloon dilation with stent placement is effective. Costamagna et al. [114] proposed progressive endoscopic dilation of the stenosis with placement of multiple stents. Patients that will benefit with endoscopic treatment are the ones diagnosed soon after surgery and have better outcome than those who develop strictures after surgery. [115] Strictures in the proximal segments of the biliary tract are more difficult to treat and require surgical treatment. [115] Davids et al. [116] performed a comparative study between surgery and endoscopic treatment, reporting similar long-term success with recurrence in 17% of patients. Percutaneos treatment require multiple sessions of balloon dilation and long-term placement of stents, [117] with morbidity associated to bleeding and bile leak up to 40%. Twenty percent of patients may eventually require redo surgery. [118]Pitt et al. [74] compared surgical repair (choledochojejunostomy vs. Hepaticojejunostomy) with percutaneous balloon dilation, reporting patency rates of 88% and 55% at 5 years for the surgical reconstruction group and percutaneous treatment.

Quality of Life

World Health Organization defines health as “a state of complete physical, mental, and social well-being, and not merely the absence of disease.”[119] Scarce information is available in the literature about Quality Of Life (QOL) after BEA. A general idea exists that patients that have a BEA will have a worst QOL; but no data is available and most information is related to surgical outcome after biliary tract reconstruction secondary to iatrogenic bile duct injury. The John Hopkins group presented a study assessing the QOL between patients who underwent surgical reconstruction of bile duct injuries and laparoscopic cholecystectomy. Their study evaluated 3 domains (Physical, psychological and social) and demonstrated lower scores in the psychological domain in patients with bile duct reconstruction ($p<0.05$). [120] Boema et al. [121] study had reduced QOL scores in the physical and mental domains; independently from the type of treatment (surgery vs. endoscopic) and the severity of the injury. De Reuver et al. [122] demonstrated a worse QOL in patients involved in litigations.

References

[1] Beal JM. Historical perspective of gallstone disease. *Surg Gynecol Obstet* 1984; 158: 181-189

[2] Hardy KJ. Carl Langenbuch and the Lazarus Hospital: events and circumstances surrounding the first cholecystectomy. *Aust N Z J Surg* 1993; 63: 56-64.

[3] van Gulik TM. Langenbuch's cholecystectomy, once a remarkably controversial operation. *Neth J Surg.* 1986; 38: 138-141.

[4] Braasch JW. Historical perspectives of biliary tract injuries. *Surg Clin North Am.* 1994; 74: 731-740.

[5] Blumgart LH. Hilar and intrahepatic biliary enteric anastomosis. *Surg Clin North Am.* 1994; 74: 845-863

[6] Gupta DK, Rohatgi M. Use of appendix in biliary atresia. *Indian J Pediatr.* 1989 Jul-Aug; 56(4):479-82.

[7] Mouret P. From the first laparoscopic cholecystectomy to the frontiers of laparoscopic surgery: the prospective futures. *Dig Surg* 1991; 8: 124.

[8] Barralet JE, Wallace LL, Strain AJ. Tissue engineering of human biliary epithelial cells on polyglycolic acid/polycaprolactone scaffolds maintains long-term phenotypic stability. *Tissue Eng.* 2003 Oct;9(5):1037-45

[9] Miyazawa M, Torii T, Toshimitsu Y, Okada K, Koyama I, Ikada Y. A tissue-engineered artificial bile duct grown to resemble the native bile duct. *Am J Transplant.* 2005 Jun;5(6):1541-7

[10] Ferraina P, Merello Laurdies J. Anastomosis biliodigestivas. Cirugía digestiva 2009; (IV); 461, pág. 1-14

[11] Buckwalter JA, Lawton RL, Tidrick RT. Bypass operation for neoplasic biliary tract obstruction. *Am J Surg* 1965: 109-100-6.

[12] Hess W, Berei G. *Textbook of Bilio-Pancreatic Diseases, pathology, diagnosis, medical treatment, surgical technique and tactics.* 1st Edition. (Vol III) PICCIN 1997, Padua, Italy.

[13] Khan T, Lwin M, Ulah S. Bilio-enteric anastomoses: Results in benign and malignant conditions. *Singapore Med J* 1993; Vol 34: 545-550.

[14] Sarfeh IJ, Rypins EB, Jakowatz JG et al. A prospective, randomized clinical investigation of cholecystoenterostomy and choledochoenterostomy. *Am J Surg* 1988; 155:411

[15] Watanapa P, Williamson RC. Surgical palliation for pancreatic cancer: developments during the past two decades. *Br J Surg* 1992; 79:8

[16] Urbach DR, Bell CM, Swanstrom LL et al. Cohort study of surgical bypass to the gallbladder or bile duct for the palliation of jaundice due to pancreatic cancer. *Ann Surg* 2003; 237:86.

[17] House MG, Choti MA. Palliative therapy for pancreatic/biliary cancer. *Surg Clin North Am* 2005; 85:359.

[18] Siquini W. *Surgical Treatment of Pancreatic Diseases.* Springer – Verlag, Italy 2009. Pg. 456.

[19] Ravindra SD, Siriwardena AK. Laparoscopic biliary bypass and current management algorithms for palliation of malignant obstructive jaundice. *Ann Surg Oncol* 2004 11:815

[20] Degenshein GA. Choledochoduodenostomy: an 18 year study of 175 consecutive cases. *Surgery.* 1974; 76:319-324.

[21] Capper WM. External choledochoduodenostomy. An evaluation of 125 cases. *Br J Surg.* 1961; 49:292-300.

[22] Wright NL. Evaluation of the results of choledochoduodenostomy. *Br J Surg.* 1968; 55:33-36.

[23] Madden JL, Chun JY, Kandalaft S, Parekh M. Choledochoduodenostomy: an unjustly maligned surgical procedure? *Am J Surg* 1970; 119:45-54.

[24] Johnson AG, Rains AJ. Prevention and treatment of recurrent bile duct stones by choledochoduodenostomy. *World J Surg*. 1978; 2:487-496.

[25] Lygidakis NJ. Choledochoduodenostomy in calculous biliary tract disease. *Br J Surg.* 1981; 68:762-765.

[26] Baker A.R et al. Sump Syndrome following choledochoduodenostomy and its Endoscopic treatment. *Br J Surg.* 1985, 72: 433-435

[27] Jones SA. et al. Sphincteroplasty in the treatment of biliary tract disease. *Surg. Clin. N. Am.* 1983, 53: 1123-37.

[28] Baker AR, Neoptolemos JP, Leese T, Fossard DP. Choledochoduodenostomy, transduodenal sphincteroplasty and sphincterotomy for calculi of the common bile duct. *Surg Gynecol Obstet.* 1987; 164:245-251.

[29] Tang CN, Siu WT, Ha JP, Li MK. Laparoscopic choledochoduodenostomy: an effective drainage procedure for recurrent pyogenic cholangitis. *Surg Endosc.* 2003; 17:1590-1594.

[30] Jeyapalan M. Almeida JA, Michaelson RL, Franklin ME Jr. Laparoscopic choledochoduodenostomy: Review of a 4 year experience with an uncommon problem. *Surg Laparosc Endosc Percutan Tech* 2002;12:148-53.

[31] Chander J, Mangla V, Vindal A, Lal P, Ramteke VK. Laparoscopic choledochoduodenostomy for biliary stone disease: a single-center 10-year experience. *J Laparoendosc Adv Surg Tech A.* 2012 Jan-Feb; 22(1):81-4.

[32] Artifon EL, Aparicio D, Paione JB, Lo SK, Bordini A, Rabello C, Otoch JP, Gupta K. Biliary drainage in patients with unresectable, malignant obstruction where ERCP fails: endoscopic ultrasonography-guided choledochoduodenostomy versus percutaneous drainage. *J Clin Gastroenterol.* 2012 Oct; 46(9):768-74.

[33] de Almeida AC, dos Santos NM, Aldeia FJ. Choledochoduodenostomy in the management of common duct stones or associated pathology—an obsolete method? *HPB Surg.* 1996; 10:27–33.

[34] Miros M, Kerlin P, Strong R, et al. Post-choledochoenterostomy "sump syndrome". *Aust N Z J Surg.* 1990;60:109–112

[35] Venerito M, Fry LC, Rickes S, et al. Cholangitis as a late complication of choledochoduodenostomy: the sump syndrome. *Endoscopy.* 2009;41(suppl 2):E142–E143

[36] Ajaz A Malik, Shiraz A Rather, Shams UL Bari and Khursheed Alam Wani. Long-term results of choledochoduodenostomy in benign biliary obstruction. *World J Gastrointest Surg.* 2012 February 27; 4(2): 36-40.

[37] Fisher J. *Mastery of Surgery.* 6th Edition. Philadelphia; USA: Lippincott Williams and Wilkins; 2012.

[38] Tang CN, Siu WT, Ha JP, Tai CK, Tsui KK, Li MK. Laparoscopic biliary bypass—a single centre experience. *Hepatogastroenterology* 2007;54:503–507.

[39] Cuschieri A, Adamson GD: Multimedia article. Laparoscopic transection choledochoduodenostomy. *Surg Endosc* 2005, 19(5):728.

[40] Marangoni G, Ali A, Faraj W, Heaton N, Rela M: Clinical features and treatment of sump syndrome following hepatico-jejunostomy. *Hepatobiliary*, 10(3):261–264.

[41] Morrissey PE, Burns GA, Cohn SM. Sump syndrome complicating Roux-en-Y hepaticojejunostomy: case report and review of the literature. *Surgery* 1996, 119(4):403–405.

[42] Suo T, Song LJ, Tong SX: Gallstone in jejunal limb with jejunocolonic fistula 10 years after Roux-en-Y choledochojejunostomy. *World J of Radiology,* 3(1):38–40.

[43] Chida T, Kageyama F, Yamada M, Yoshii S, Honjo Y, Takai T, Iwaoka Y, Terai T, Kagami T, Yamazaki S *et al.* A case of hemorrhage from varices of an interposed jejunum after choledochojejunostomy treated successfully by endoscopic injection using alpha-cyanoacrylate monomer. *Nippon Shokakibyo Gakkai Zasshi* 1661, 107(10):1661–1668.

[44] Leppard WM, Shary TM, Adams DB and Morgan K. Choledochoduodenostomy: Is It Really So Bad? *J Gastrointest Surg* 2011; 15 (5) 754-7

[45] Clavien PA. *Atlas of upper gastrointestinal and hepato-pancreato-biliary surgery*. New York: Springer; 2007.

[46] Fletcher DR, Hobbs MST, Tan P, et al: Complications of cholecystectomy: Risks of the laparoscopic approach and protective effects of operative cholangiography. A population-based study. *Ann Surg* 229:449-457, 1999

[47] Sarmiento J. Hepaticojejunostomy: Indications and Surgical Technique. *Operative Techniques in General Surgery,* Vol 2, No 4 (December), 2000: pp 295-303

[48] Diao M, Li L, Cheng W. Laparoscopic versus Open Roux-en-Y hepatojejunostomy for children with choledochal cysts: intermediate-term follow-up results. *Surg Endosc.* 2011 May; 25(5):1567-73.
[49] Hepp J, Couinaud C. L´abord et l´utilisation du canal hepatique dans le reparations de la voie biliare principale. *Presse Med* 1956; 64: 947
[50] Guglielmi A, Ruzzenente A, Iacono C. *Surgical Treatment of Hilar and Intrahepatic Cholangiocarcinoma.* Springer-Verlag Italia 2008.
[51] Myburgh JA. The Hepp-Couinaud Approach to Strictures of the Bile Ducts I. Injuries, Choledochal Cysts,and Pancreatitis. *Annals of Surgery* 1993; Vol. 218, No. 5, 615-620.
[52] Singhal D, van Gulik TM, Gouma DJ. Palliative management of hilar cholangiocarcinoma. *Surg Oncol* 2005; 14(2):59–74
[53] Connors S, Wigmore SJ, Madhavan KK et al. Surgical palliation for unresectable hilar cholangiocarcinoma. *HPB Surg* 2005; 7:273–277.
[54] Tochi A, Costa G, Lepre L, et al. The long-term outcome of hepaticojejunostomy in the Treatment of bening bile duct strictures. *Ann Surg* 1996; 224(2): 162-167.
[55] Traverso LW. The Longmire I, II, and III operations. *Am J Surg.* 2003 May, Volume 185, Issue 5
[56] Winslow E, Fialkowski E, Linehan D, Hawkins W, Picus D, Strasberg S. “Sideways”: Results of Repair of Biliary Injuries Using a Policy of Side-To-Side Hepatico-Jejunostomy. Ann Surg, Vol 249 (3): 2009; 426-434.
[57] Mercado MA, Chan C, Orozco H, Cano-Gutiérrez G, Chaparro JM, Galindo E, Vilatobá M, Samaniego-Arvizu G. To stent or not to stent bilioenteric anastomosis after iatrogenic injury: a dilemma not answered? Arch Surg 2002; 137: 60-63
[58] De Ledinghen VPerson BLegoux JL et al. Prevention of biliary stent occlusion by ursodeoxycholic acid plus norfloxacin: a multicenter randomized trial. *Dig Dis Sci.*2000;45145- 150
[59] Zafar S, Rizwan M, Raza R, N Khan M, Kasi M. Early complications after biliary enteric anastomosis for benign diseases: A retrospective analysis. *BMC Surgery* 2011, 11:19.
[60] Hall JG, Pappas TN. Current management of biliary strictures. *J Gastrointest Surg* 2004; 8: 1098-1110.
[61] Ahrendt SA, Pitt HA. Surgical therapy of iatrogenic lesions of biliary tract. *World J Surg* 2001; 25: 1360-1365.
[62] Sicklick JK, Camp MS, Lillemoe KD, Melton GB, Yeo CJ, Campbell KA, Talamini MA, Pitt HA, Coleman J, Sauter PA, Cameron JL. Surgical management of bile duct injuries sustained during laparoscopic

cholecystectomy: perioperative results in 200 patients. *Ann Surg* 2005; 241: 786-792; discussion 793-795.

[63] Tocchi A, Mazzoni G, Liotta G, Lepre L, Cassini D, Miccini M. Late development of bile duct cancer in patients who had biliary-enteric study of more than 1,000 patients. *Ann Surg* 2001, 234(2):210-214.

[64] Lillemoe KD, Melton GB, Cameron JL, Pitt HA, Campbell KA, Talamini MA, Sauter PA, Coleman J, Yeo CJ. Postoperative bile duct strictures: management and outcome in the 1990s. *Ann Surg* 2000; 232: 430-441.

[65] McDonald ML, Farnell MB, Nagorney DM, Ilstrup DM, Kutch JM. Benign biliary strictures: repair and outcome with a contemporary approach. *Surgery* 1995; 118: 582-590; discussion 590-591.

[66] Shimizu T, Yoshida H, Mamada Y, Taniai N, Matsumoto S, Mizuguchi Y, Yokomuro S, Arima Y, Akimaru K, Tajiri T. Postoperative bile leakage managed successfully by intrahepatic biliary ablation with ethanol. *World J Gastroenterol* 2006 June 7; 12(21): 3450-3452.

[67] Kapoor S, Nundy S. Bile Duct Leaks from the Intrahepatic Biliary Tree: A Review of Its Etiology, Incidence, and Management. *HPB Surgery* 2012, Article ID 752932

[68] Mongestern L, Berci G, Pasternak E. Bile leakage after biliary tract surgery. A laparoscopic perspective. *Surg Endosc* 1993; 7: 432-438.

[69] Kapoor V, Baron R, Peterson M. Bile Leaks After Surgery. *AJR* 2004; 182:451–458.

[70] Pecchi A, De Santis M, Gibertini, Tarantino G, Gerunda G, Torricelli P, Di Benedetto F. Role of Magnetic Resonance Imaging in the Detection of Anastomotic Biliary Strictures After Liver Transplantation. *Transplantation Proceedings* 2011; 43, 1132–1135.

[71] Katz LH, Benjaminov O, Belinki A, Geler A, Braun M, Knizhnik M, Aizner S, Shaharabani E, Sulkes J, Shabtai E, Pappo O, Atar E, Tur-Kaspa R, Mor E, Ben-Ari Z. Magnetic resonance cholangiopancreatography for the accurate diagnosis of biliary complications after liver transplantation: comparison with endoscopic retrograde cholangiography and percutaneous transhepatic cholangiography – long-term follow-up. *Clin Transplant* 2010: 24: E163–E169.

[72] Beltrán MM, Marugán RB, Oton E, Blesa C, Nun˜o J. Accuracy of magnetic resonance cholangiography in the evaluation of late biliary complications after orthotopic liver transplantation. *Transplant Proc* 2005: 7: 3924.

[73] Cantwell C, Pena C, Gervais D, Hahn P, Dawson S, Mueller P. Thirty Years' Experience with Balloon Dilation of Benign Postoperative Biliary Strictures: Long-term Outcomes. *Radiology* 2008 (3): 249.

[74] Pitt HA, Kaufman SL, Coleman J, White RI, Cameron JL. Benign postoperative biliary strictures: operate or dilate? Ann Surg 1989; 210:417–425.

[75] Williams HJ, Bender CE, May GR. Benign postoperative biliary strictures: dilation with fluoroscopic guidance. *Radiology* 1987; 163: 629–634.

[76] Mueller PR, vanSonnenberg E, Ferrucci JT, et al. Biliary stricture dilation: multicenter review of clinical management in 73 patients. *Radiology* 1986; 160:17–22.

[77] Oishi AJ, Sarr MG, Nagorney DM, Traynor MD. Long-Term Outcome of Cholecystoenterostomy as a Definitive Biliary Drainage Procedure for Benign Disease. *World J. Surg* 1995; 19: 616-620, 1995.

[78] Thomson SR. Sequelae of cholecystojejunostomy for benign intrapancreatic biliary strictures. *S Afr Surg* 1998;36(1):26–29.

[79] Porter DH, Kim D, Austin RM. Cholecystojejunostomy Intussusception. *Gastrointest Radiol* 13:227-229 (1988).

[80] Carpenter S, Brown KA. Chronic complications after cholecystojejunostomy. *Am J Gastroenterol* 1994; 89: 2073-2075.

[81] Miller JT Jr, De Odorico I, Marx MV. Cholecystojejunostomy varices demonstrated by enteroclysis. *Abdom Imaging* 1997;22: 474-476.

[82] Salam AA, Goldman M, Smith D, et al. Gastric, intestinal, and gallbladder varices: hemodynamic and therapeutic considerations. *South Med* J 1979; 72:402–408.

[83] Pilgrim CHC, Satgunaseelan L, Ward SM, Evans PM. Gallbladder Carcinoma as a Long-Term Complication of Cholecystojejunostomy. *J Gastrointest Surg* (2009) 13:2330–2332.

[84] Malik AA, Rather S, Bari S, Wani KA. Long-term results of choledochoduodenostomy in benign biliary obstruction. *World J Gastrointest Surg* 2012 February 27; 4(2): 36-40.

[85] de Aretxabala X, Bahamondes JC. Choledochoduodenostomy for common bile duct stones. *World J Surg.* 1998; 22:1171.

[86] Panis Y, Fagniez PL, Brisset D, Lacaine F, Levard H, Hay JM. Long term results of choledochoduodenostomy versus choledochojejunostomy for choledocholithiasis. The French Association for Surgical Research. *Surg Gynecol Obstet.* 1993 Jul; 177(1):33-7.

[87] Gupta BS. Choledochoduodenostomy: a study of 28 consecutive cases. *Kathmandu University Medical Journal* (2003) Vol. 2, No. 3, Issue7, 193 – 197.

[88] LING Xiao-feng, XU Zhi, WANG Li-xin, HOU Chun-sheng, XIU Dian-rong, ZHANG Tong-lin and ZHOU Xiao-si. Long-term outcomes of choledochoduodenostomy for hepatolithiasis. *Chinese Medical Journal* 2010; 123(2):137-141.

[89] Khajanchee YS, Cassera MA, Hammill CW, Swanström L, Hansen P. Outcomes Following Laparoscopic Choledochoduodenostomy in the Management of Benign Biliary Obstruction. *J Gastrointest Surg* (2012) 16:801–805.

[90] De Almeida A, Cruz A, Aldeia F. Side to side choledochodenostomy in the management of cholelithiasis and associated disease: facts and fiction. *American Journal of Surgery* 1984; 147: 253–259.

[91] Baker A, Neoptolemos J, Leese T et al. Long term follow-up of patients with side to side choledochoduodenostomy and transduodenal sphincteroplasty. *Annals of the Royal College of Surgeons of England.* 1987; 68: 253–257.

[92] Qadan M, Clarke S, Morrow S, Triadafilopoulos G, Visser B. Sump Syndrome as a Complication of Choledochoduodenostomy. *Dig Dis Sci* (2012) 57:2011–2015

[93] Caroli-Bosc FX, Demarquay JF, Peten EP, et al. Endoscopic management of sump syndrome after choledochoduodenostomy: retrospective analysis of 30 cases. *Gastrointest Endosc.* 2000; 51:180.

[94] Siegel JH. Duodenoscopic sphincterotomy in the treatment of the ''sump syndrome''. *Dig Dis Sic.* 1981; 26:922.

[95] Hallstone A, Triadafilopoulos G. Spontaneous sump syndrome: successful treatment by duodenoscopic sphincterotomy. *Am J Gastroenterol.* 1990; 85:1518.

[96] Marbet UA, Stalder GA, Faust H, Harder F, Gyr K. Endoscopic sphincterotomy and surgical approaches in the treatment of the 'sump syndrome'. *Gut.* 1987; 28:142.

[97] Eleftheriadis E, Tzioufa V, Kotzampassi K, Aletras H. Common bile duct mucosa in choledochoduodenostomy patients— histological and histochemical study. *HPB Surg.* 1988; 1:15–20.

[98] Nakamura Y, Ohta G, Nagakawa T, Matsubara F. Pathological findings of hepatolithiasis. *Jpn J Gastroenterol.* 1981; 78:874–882.

[99] Komi N, Tamura T, Tsuge S, et al. Relation of patient age to premalignant alterations in choledochal cyst epithelium. *J Pediatr Surg.* 1986; 21:430–433.

[100] Rothlin MA, Lopfe M and Largiader F. Long-Term Results of Hepaticojejunostomy for Benign Lesions of the Bile Ducts. *The American Journal of Surgery.* 1998; 1: 22–25.

[101] Ross CB, H'Doubler WZ, Sharp KW et al. Recent experience with benign biliary strictures. *American Surgeon.* 1989; 1: 64–70.

[102] Schmidt SC, Langrehr JM, Hintze RE, Neuhaus P. Long-term results and risk factors influencing outcome of major bile duct injuries following cholecystectomy. *Br J Surg* 2005; 92:76–82.

[103] Mercado MÁ, Franssen B. Transition from a low: to a high-volume centre for bile duct repair: changes in technique and improved outcome. *HPB* 2011; 13:767–773.

[104] House M, Cameron J, Schulick R. Incidence and outcome of biliary strictures after pancreaticoduodenectomy. *Annals of Surgery* 2006 vol. 243, no. 5, pp. 571–576.

[105] Kucukay F, Okten R, Yurdakul M, Ozdemir E, Erat S, Parlak E, Disibeyaz S, Ozer I, Bostanci EB, Olcer T, Tola M. Long-term Results of Percutaneous Biliary Balloon Dilation Treatment for Benign Hepaticojejunostomy Strictures: Are Repeated Balloon Dilations Necessary? *J Vasc Interv Radiol* 2012; 23:1347–1355.

[106] Pitt HA, Miyamoto T, Parapatis SK, Tompkins RK, Longmire WP Jr. Factors influencing outcome in patients with postoperative biliary strictures. *Am J Surg* 1982; 144:14–21.

[107] Pellegrini CA, Thomas MJ, Way LW. Recurrent biliary stricture. Patterns of recurrence and outcome of surgical therapy. *Am J Surg* 1984; 147:175–180.

[108] de Castro S, Kuhlmann K, Busch O, van Delden O, Lameris J, van Gulik T, Obertop H, Gouma D. Incidence and management of biliary leakage after hepaticojejunostomy. *J Gastrointest Surg* 2005;9:1163–1173.

[109] Lillemoe KD, Martin SA, Cameron JL, Yeo CJ, Talamini MA, Kaushal S, Coleman J, Venbrux AC, Savader SJ, Osterman FA, Pitt HA. Major bile duct injuries during laparoscopic cholecystectomy. Follow-up after combined surgical and radiologic management. Ann Surg 1997; 225: 459-468; discussion 468-471.

[110] Terblanche J, Worthley CS, Spence RA, Krige JE. High or low hepaticojejunostomy for bile duct strictures? Surgery 1990; 108: 828-834.

[111] Rege RV. Adverese effects of biliary obstruction: Implications for treatment of patients with obstructive jaundice. AJR 1995; 164: 287-93.

[112] Schmidt SC, Langrehr JM, Hintze RE, Neuhaus P. Longterm results and risk factors influencing outcome of major bile duct injuries following cholecystectomy. *Br J Surg* 2005; 92:76-82.

[113] Bauer TW, Morris FB, Lowenstein A, et al. The consequences of major bile duct injury during laparoscopic cholecystectomy. *J Gastrointest Surg* 1998; 2: 61-66.

[114] Costamagna G, Pandolfi M, Mutignani M, Spada C, Perri V. Long-term results of endoscopic management of postoperative bile duct strictures with increasing numbers of stents. *Gastrointest Endosc.* 2001;54:162–168.

[115] Jacques J. G. H. M. Bergman, Lotje Burgemeister, Marco J. Bruno, Erik A. J. Rauws, Dirk J. Gouma, Guido N. J. Tytga, Kees Huibregtse. Long-term follow-up after biliary stent placement for postoperative bile duct stenosis. *Gastrointestinal endoscopy* 2001; (54): 154-161.

[116] Davids PH, Tanka AK, Rauws EA, van Gulik TM, van Leeuwen DJ, de Wit LT, et al. Benign biliary strictures. Surgery or endoscopy? *Ann Surg* 1993; 217:237-43.

[117] Jan YY, Chen MF, Hung CF. Balloon dilatation of intrahepatic duct and biliary-enteric anastomosis strictures. Long term results. *Int Surg* 1994;79:103-5.

[118] Vos PM, van Beek EJ, Smits NJ, Rauws EA, Gouma DJ,Reeders JW. Percutaneous balloon dilatation for benign hepaticojejunostomy strictures. *Abdom Imaging* 2000; 25 :134-8.

[119] Preamble to the Constitution of the World Health Organization as adopted by the International Health Conference, New York, 19–22 June, 1946; signed on 22 July 1946 by the representatives of 61 States (Official Records of the World Health Organization, no. 2, p. 100) and entered into force on 7 April 1948.

[120] Melton GB, Lillemoe KD, Cameron JL, Sauter PA, Coleman J, Yeo CJ. Major bile duct injuries associated with laparoscopic cholecystectomy: Effect of surgical repair on quality of life. *Annals of surgery* 2002; 235:888-895.

[121] Boerma D, Rauws EAJ, Keulemans YLA, et al. Impaired quality of life 5 years after bile duct injury during the laparoscopic cholecystectomy: A prospective analysis. *Ann Surg* 2001; 234:750–757.

[122] deReuver P, Sprangers M, Rauws E, et al. Impact of bile duct injury after laparoscopic cholecystectomy on quality of life: a longitudinal study after multidisciplinary treatment. *Endoscopy* 2008;40(8):637–43.

In: Anastomoses ISBN: 978-1-62618-657-6
Editors: F. King, McKineley A. Malloy © 2013 Nova Science Publishers, Inc.

Chapter II

Intestinal Anastomosis Education and Training

José C. Manuel-Palazuelos, Federico Castillo, Carlos Gavilanes, Manuel Gómez-Fleitas and Juan C. Rodríguez-Sanjuán

Department of General Surgery, University Hospital Marqués de Valdecilla, University of Cantabria, Santander, Spain

Abstract

The aim of a gastro-intestinal suture is to provide a hermetic closure in the intestine or in an anastomosis.

To achieve a successful suture, a proper technique is essential, with strict adherence to surgical principles, such as suture tension, border vascularization and intestinal diameter. Also the patient biological condition has to be considered. All of these factors influence suture healing but the experience and skill of the surgeon are probably most important in the final outcome of the anastomosis.

Until recently the learning of any surgical procedure was based on direct operation on the patient, with initial supervision by an experienced surgeon. This has several drawbacks such as risks for the patient, long learning curves and an increase in operating room costs because of greater operation times. Laparoscopic procedures need even longer and more complex training periods due to the lack of tactile sensation and two-dimension view. The problem is even greater in the case of residents who are less experienced in surgery in general. To speed up learning and avoid direct training on patients, training laboratories have been designed, where physical and virtual reality simulators can be used.

The usefulness of training using simulation in basic surgical techniques has been shown in improving general surgical skills and performance of intestinal anastomosis with synthetic materials. Training in intestinal anastomosis using dead animal viscera is very similar to the clinical setting and has advantages over other options such as live animals, simulators or corpses. The training on live animals reproduces real clinical settings although it has drawbacks such as high costs or the sacrifice of the animal. Cadaver surgery is also very similar to real clinical settings but is hardly available. Virtual reality is very different from real clinical settings and evidence for validation of most designed devices is lacking. These models could be used as the first contact with laparoscopic training, according to the conclusions of the systematic reviews published to date. However, the advantage in resident training with some laparoscopic experience has not been shown. On the other hand these systems are expensive, although less so than direct training on patients.

As a result, the aim of this work is to expose which is the best training method in every anastomosis type and the influence that the different simulators or training with animals have on learning surgical skills.

Introduction

Postgraduate training in surgery lasts currently 5 or more years after graduation. Such teaching occurs in hospital based residency programs [1]. The concept of surgical residency in a hospital is attributed to William S. Halsted which was one of his first achievements at The Johns Hopkins Hospital. He designed a training program for surgeons based primarily on the German, Austrian, and Swiss models. The Germanic system of training for young surgeons consisted of assistants spending many years in a university surgical clinic who eventually achieved the position of first assistant to the professor. Halsted introduced a system in which the medical school graduates entered into a university sponsored, hospital-based surgical training program that, over a several-year period of increasing responsibility, slowly led to the training of young surgeons who were well versed in anatomy, pathology, bacteriology, and physiology.

The training program culminated in a final period of near-total independence and autonomous activity. This eventually made the surgical residency training programs as we know them today [2, 3]. Surgical training has undergone dramatic changes in recent years. Knowledge development and new technologies have led to the gradual increase in the surgical therapeutic arsenal, so that the general surgeon extensively trained, able to treat a wide variety of processes in multiple organ systems, has become a rarity. Over the past 30 years, general surgery has given way to several subspecialties [1].

For many procedures, the observed associations between hospital volume and operative mortality are largely mediated by surgeon volume. Patients can often substantially improve their chances of survival, even in high-volume hospitals, by selecting surgeons who perform the operations frequently. The key mechanism could simply be "practical" clinical judgment and technical skill that are achieved only by surgeons who perform a specific procedure with sufficient frequency [4].

Currently, many graduate residents in general surgery choose to receive additional training in a subspecialty, before starting independent exercise. Many residents, particularly in university hospital and reference system programs, contact almost exclusively with subspecialists during their residence. Since more interventions are performed by young specialists after residency training and fellowships, the training achieved during the residence becomes increasingly less complete. Consequently, many residents believe that training in general surgery in the current format does not prepare them properly for practice, and therefore they feel compelled to find additional training. There is now a generalized concept among members of the profession, that graduates in residency programs are not as capable as those of a generation ago [1].

Until recently, learning surgical procedure was based on the operation realization, initially monitored, on the patients themselves. This implies a long learning curve with increased morbidity, and possibly mortality, and worse long-term outcomes [5]. Today the residents are much more supervised and have less exposure to the operating room environment. Also, current trainees have less independent surgical experience because of pressures for greater operating room efficiencies and the shorter workweek for residents due to the introduction of European directives on working time seeking the conciliation of work and family life. All of these have led to a reassessment of training methods [6, 7, 8].

Much of the problem of inexperience could be solved by simulating clinical scenarios. Residents could learn technical skills and gain experience in decision-making models, in safe simulated environments but the clinical simulation tools today remain relatively expensive and under development.

Nevertheless, simulation promises to transform completely surgical education in the years ahead [1].

The ability to acquire surgical skills requires consistent practice, and evidence suggests that many of these technical skills can be learned out of the operating theater [9, 10, 11, 12]. Surgical simulation offers the opportunity for trainees to practice their surgical skills prior to entering the operating room, allowing detailed feedback and objective assessment of their performance. This enables better patient safety and standards of care. Surgical simulators can be divided into organic or inorganic types. Organic simulators, consisting of live animal and fresh human cadaver models, are considered to be of high-fidelity. Inorganic types comprise virtual reality simulators and synthetic bench models. Current evidence suggests that skills acquired through training with simulators positively transfers to the clinical setting and improves operative outcome. The major challenge for the future revolves around understanding the value of this new technology and developing an educational curriculum that can incorporate surgical simulators [13].

While there may be compelling reasons to reduce reliance on patients, cadavers, and animals for surgical training, none of the methods of simulated training (including computer simulation) has yet been shown to be better than other forms of surgical training. In addition, little is known about the real costs (including adverse outcomes in patients) of either simulated or standard surgical training [14].

Manually and Stapled Bowel Anastomosis

Within the past 200 years, gastrointestinal anastomosis has been transformed from a dangerous venture into a safe and routinely performed procedure. Among these advances was the transition to scientifically-based medicine, chiefly the knowledge of the importance of serosa apposition introduced by Lembert [15]. The French physician and surgeon Antoine Thomas Alfred Étienne Lembert, born April 19, 1802 in Nancy and died in Paris of a stomach cancer at the age of 49 in 1851 is worth mentioning [16]. In 1826 Lembert developed a suture technique using interrupted sutures that passed through the entire bowel wall except for the mucous membrane [17]. Later in 1887, Halsted described that the submucosa provides most of the tensile strength to the gastro-intestinal tract. The bulk of collagen is contained within this layer, along with blood vessels, lymphatics, and nerve fibres. For this reason he altered Lembert's suture technique, passing the needle through the submucosa but not into the bowel lumen [18]. Other suture patterns carry no less important eponyms such as Cushing's suture: A type of variation on continuous mattress sutures. The suture starts with Lembert's technique and, after knotting, the bites are taken parallel to wound edges alternately on either side to the end. The suture runs parallel to the wound edges through the tissue and the exposed part of the suture runs perpendicular to the wound edges. The submucosa is engaged but not the mucosa. Connell's suture is similar to Cushing's except that complete penetration into the bowel lumen is performed.

An additional modern advance in bowel anastomosis has been the advent of staplers, although the Murphy Button device described in 1892 was the first popular stapling prototype [19, 20]. Surgical stapling devices were first introduced by Hültl in 1908, although they did not gain popularity then or for some time afterwards because the early instruments were cumbersome and unreliable. Further progress was not remarkable until the early 1960's when the Institute for Experimental Apparatus and Instruments in Moscow developed a group of instruments capable of performing gastrointestinal tract anastomosis [21].

Anastomotic Healing

The process of intestinal anastomotic healing is similar to wound healing elsewhere in the body and can be divided into (A) acute inflammatory - lag - phase, (B) proliferative phase, and (C) remodelling or maturation phase. Collagen is the single most important molecule for determining intestinal wall strength, which makes its metabolism of particular interest for understanding anastomotic healing. A critical stage in collagen formation is the hydroxylation of proline during the maturation phase to hydroxyproline, which gives the molecule its structural strength. The bursting pressure of an anastomosis is often used to gauge the strength of the healing process. This pressure has been found to increase rapidly in the early postoperative period, reaching 60% of the strength of the surrounding bowel within three to four days and 100% in one week [22, 23]. We cannot forget the serosa on the bowel wall which also influences the ease with which both ends of the intestine may be joined. This effect is emphasized by the increased technical difficulty of joining extraperitoneal bowel ends, for example the thoracic esophagus and the rectum.

Factors Associated with Anastomotic Failure

Complications associated with anastomotic breakdown increase morbidity and mortality. Reported failure rates range from 1 to 24%, depending on what type of anastomosis was performed and whether the operation was scheduled or emergent [24]. Signs and symptoms suggesting postoperative anastomotic leak appear usually between days four and seven, and include abdominal pain or peritonitis, often leading to a systemic inflammatory response syndrome (SIRS) and sepsis.

Factors contributing to anastomotic failure may be local or systemic. Among the systemic factors are malnutrition, vitamin deficiencies, anemia, diabetes mellitus, uremia, sepsis, previous irradiation or chemotherapy, steroid use, certain disorders such as Crohn's disease - which is associated with poor anastomotic healing and increased anastomotic leak rates [25, 26], smoking and heavy alcohol consumption [27], or hypothermia [28].

Among the local factors, blood flow is a critical factor in tissue healing. The increased vascularity of the bowel wall is the reason why gastric and small bowel anastomoses heal more rapidly than anastomoses involving the esophagus or the large bowel. In preparing the bowel ends for anastomosis, it is imperative that the mesentery be handled carefully and to preserve vascularization. Prevention of tension at the anastomosis is also critical. Inverting the cut bowel edges in colorectal surgery is also important [29]. Bowel preparation may not be essential and it may actually be harmful. A Finnish randomized prospective study published in 2000 first suggested that patients with bowel preparation had no influence on leak, infection, or restoration of bowel function rates [30]. Subsequent studies have showed that rates of both anastomotic leakage and wound infection were actually significantly higher in patients receiving bowel preparation compared to those who did not [31]. This may be related to the change in native intestinal flora after bowel preparation.

In practice the choice of anastomosis may be influenced by the diameter of the bowel ends, edema, accessibility and site of anastomosis, contamination, available time and equipment and underlying pathology. Anastomoses can be described as follows: sutured: (1) interrupted or continuous; (2) one or two-layer; (3) end-to-end or side-to-side (or any combination); (4) various suture materials; (5) extramucosal or full thickness sutures; and (6) size of and spacing between each suture; and stapled: (1) side-to-side or end-to-end (or any combination); (2) staple lines oversewn, buried or not; and (3) various stapling devices [32].

What does the evidence say on the topic? Prospective, randomized trials have not demonstrated any differences between stapled and hand-sewn anastomosis in terms of leakage rates, length of hospital stay, or overall morbidity [33].

In 2007 the Cochrane Collaboration published a meta-analysis of randomized controlled trials regarding ileocolic anastomoses. A stapled side-to-side anastomosis is recommended following a right hemicolectomy, particularly if this operation is performed for a colonic adenocarcinoma [34]. Most evidence currently favors a stapled side-to-side ileocolic anastomosis in Crohn's disease [35] or suggests that suturing and stapling are equivalents [36]. No evidence favors sutured end-to-end anastomosis. In contrast, level 1a evidence has shown that sutured or endoluminal circular stapled techniques are equally suitable for colorectal anastomoses [37].

In trauma patients, level 3 currently remains our best available evidence, and suggests that stapled small bowel anastomoses may be best avoided in trauma [38, 39]. The question of stapled colonic anastomosis remains uncertain.

Training According to Surgical Approach

Open Approach

Intestinal anastomosis is one of the most important and frequent procedures in clinical practice of a surgeon. As a result, a proper performance is needed and the best way to achieve this is adequate training before undertaking anastomoses in the patient. Despite the recent technological advances and the development of laparoscopic and robotic-assisted surgery, training in open surgery must not be underestimated since it is the base to start any type of surgical training as well as the last resort in case of trouble when operating on laparoscopically.

Bench training is advisable before starting clinical practice. Learning curves are shortened since the techniques can be repeated many times, which could take months or years or be virtually impossible in the clinical ground. The abilities acquired by means of simulation can be transferred to the operating room. As a result, simulation-based training is the ideal tool to increase patient safety and to correct the lack of clinical experience as well as coordination failures of the multidisciplinary team [6]. Any type of surgical training should start by the open approach. In the case of intestinal anastomosis, it is necessary to know the basic techniques and maneuvers, such as the different types of stitches, knots and anastomoses. Then, attention should be paid to the handling of the abdominal wall. Finally, specific training on anastomosis can be started to avoid the complications seen in clinical practice, many as a result of technical errors [40]. Virtually every anastomosis type can be, currently, susceptible of training. The most used models are the pig intestine *ex-vivo* and the pig or sheep *in-vivo*. The *ex-vivo* model allows practicing mainly entero-enteric, gastro-jejunal and ileo-colic anastomosis. This model provides better control of the setting for the initial anastomosis training since it allows placing the intestinal segments as needed. Its main inconvenience is tissue conservation damage, which occasionally makes wall layer differentiation more difficult. For this reason, a good model for beginners is the gastro-jejunal anastomosis since the gastric wall is wider.

In-vivo models allow more types of anastomoses and even more complex, such as esophago-gastric, low and ultralow colo-rectal and colo-anal anastomosis, in a biological and anatomic setting similar to a real operation.

In this phase of the training, attention must be paid to the teaching of manual anastomosis, more technically demanding and dependant on the human factor. As a result, more training is needed.

The teaching procedure we do begins with the watching of videos with the technique to learn and a description by an expert of the essential steps and technical details. Then, the trainee begins making side-to-side anastomoses in different viscuses in an *ex-vivo* model.

For the training of side-to-side anastomoses, the two intestines are placed in parallel and joined by two stitches at both ends. Then, a seromuscular suture (either with running or interrupted stitches) is carried out in the posterior surface of the future anastomosis. The intestines are opened and another suture is started in the middle, including the entire wall of both bowels. The suture progresses to one corner. At this point a Connell's stitch is done: when the needle is inside the intestinal lumen, it is passed outside into the same intestine side; then, in the other bowel the needle is passed out-to-in and then in-to-out (Figure 1). This Connell's stitch must be repeated in the other intestine by new movements out-to-in and then in-to-out to allow the needle to be well placed to begin the suture on the anterior surface of the anastomosis (Figure 2). The distance between the needle passes must be short to prevent the initial stitch remaining hidden. With a second thread, another suture is also started in the middle of the posterior surface, going to the opposite side. At the corner, Connell's stitch is also done, and upon anastomosis completion, both threads are tied in the middle of the anterior anastomosis surface.

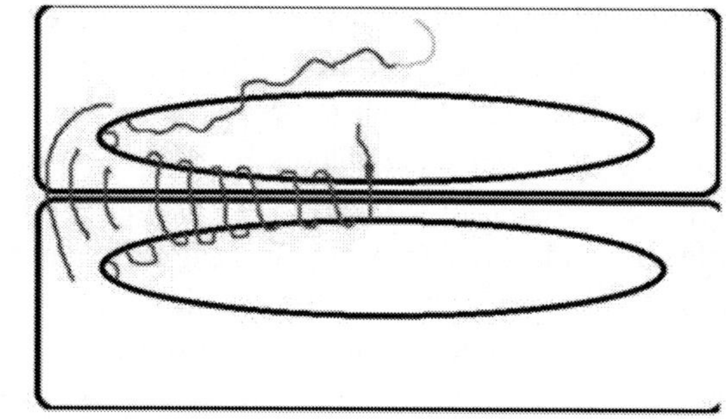

Figure 1.

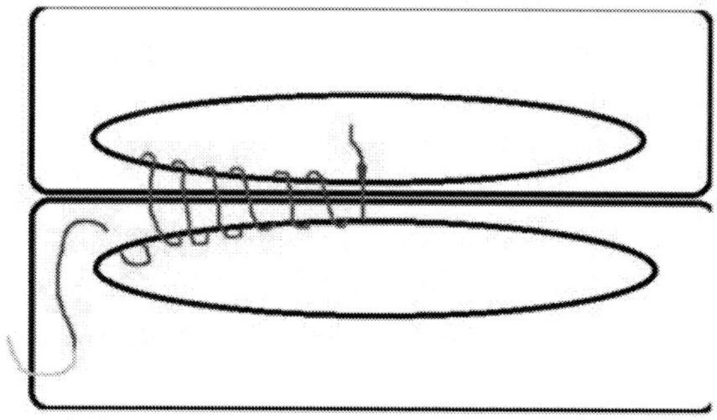

Figure 2.

In this phase, training with staplers can also be done in esophago-gastric, low colo-rectal and esophago-jejunal anastomoses, which are frequently used in clinical practice. They are especially difficult anastomoses, with a high risk of failure for anatomic reasons. As a result it is important to train on them to minimize technical errors when they have to be done in the real patient.

Laparoscopic Approach

This approach produces important perception changes in the surgeon. Vision is in two dimensions and the touch sensation is lacking so the consistency transmitted from the tissues is much decreased. Specific training must therefore be done in laparoscopic techniques. The essentials of the open techniques are the same, although adapted to the laparoscopic instruments and some movement limitations. Some threads have "memory" and are more difficult to manage, especially in small spaces. The needle is also hard to manage, first due to the difficulty of properly placing it in the tip of the needle-holder and second, because of precision loss due to holder length. This could be a cause of lesions in the abdominal structures. Today some three-dimension equipment is available which facilitates vision, increases depth perception and, therefore, surgical precision, although specific training is also needed.

Another problem found in laparoscopy is fatigue due to the demanding positions the surgeon has to adopt. Ergonomics is, therefore, another suggestion for improvement, especially in anastomosis training, since they are demanding techniques with high concentration necessity which can be disturbed because of bad positions or use of poor ergonomic instruments. As a result, not only does the technique itself need to be trained in but also the way to do it to avoid surgeon lesions and increase efficacy.

There are some specific laparoscopic instruments to make manual anastomosis, such as the Endo Stitch™ device (Covidien Surgical) and dentate threads, which help suture performance.

However, due to greater complexity of manual techniques, with intracorporeal knots and ergonomic problems, stapled anastomoses - less influenced by the surgeon - are preferred in many laparoscopic procedures. The available laparoscopic staplers allow performing any type of intestinal anastomosis.

For an adequate training in laparoscopy, successive phases with increasing complexity are needed, since the learning curve is longer than in open surgery. The training should begin in the endotrainer and, then, should continue in *in-vivo* models. Some difficult anastomoses, such as the low-rectal type, ought to be complemented with training on cadavers, the most realistic model [41].

Robotic-Assisted Techniques

Robotic-assisted surgery shares most features with laparoscopic surgery with the main advantage of higher precision. This is due to more intuitive movements of the instruments, movement scale, tremor suppression, increased ambidexterity, three-dimension vision and, most importantly, the ability to imitate human wrist movements with the possibility of 360° rotation. This greatly facilitates surgical work, increasing skills with better ergonomics and, therefore, making manual anastomoses easier in cases where conventional laparoscopy would be very limited. The main disadvantages of robotic-assisted surgery are high costs, big size of the equipment and limited surgical range [42]. Also, the robot does not currently have adaptors for staplers, so they have to be introduced by the assistant surgeon, who occasionally has trouble doing so due to the trocar placement and even to the robot arms.

Intestinal Anastomoses: Need for Laboratory Training

In the mid XIX century Halsted and other surgeons thought that the learning method consisted of watching, doing and teaching. An expert surgeon, as Halsted was, taught colleagues or fellows surgical techniques in the operating-room - even those he designed himself - for intestinal anastomosis, such as the U-shaped stitch. Other surgeons like Lembert, Cushing or Connell follow the same principles and also designed intestinal suture techniques, with the aim of performing hermetic anastomosis, with little tissue damage and therefore, low stenosis and leak rates.

In those years there was already important controversy concerning which technique was best: one or two layers, interrupted or running suture. Halsted highlighted the advantages of one layer for gastro-intestinal sutures, since he thought that the two layers technique was harmful because it was considered more traumatic, slower, more expensive and predisposing to stenosis.

Nowadays, evidence concerning the superiority of one layer running suture is lacking [18]. The higher speed during performance makes this the most accepted technique although surgical societies do not opt for any particular suture type.

By the end of the XX century, the anastomosis techniques had become standardized. New materials arrived (Polyglactin, Polyglactin 910, polydioxanona), which allowed easy handling and reabsorbing several months later, thus favoring the development of running suture [43, 44, 45]. Also, at the end of the XX century manufacturers developed a variety of devices –staplers- which made it possible to perform automatic anastomosis. Clinical studies have shown lower leak rates, especially when dealing with high risk anastomoses such as those located in the esophagus or rectum [34]. As a result, staplers became extensively used in most hospitals, also under the influence of manufacturers.

Progress on surgery and the birth and development of laparoscopy have meant that surgical techniques such as intestinal anastomoses, apparently consolidated, need revision as well as teaching methods, considering the different conditions of the laparoscopic view. This is even more important due to the time restriction on residents in operating-rooms. As a result, training laboratories become decisive in training in surgical techniques.

In the beginning of laparoscopy, the surgeon had to adapt to the new conditions but using manual techniques, leading to a combination of anastomoses performed through laparoscopic and open approaches. This is the case of colectomy or gastrectomy where the anastomoses, either stapled or hand-performed, were extracorporeal, although the increasing demand of less invasive surgery favors intracorporeal anastomosis. These are more technically demanding and, therefore, there is a need for more complex training [46].

On the other hand residents nowadays spend less time in operating-rooms than before, have more complex techniques to learn (due to laparoscopic surgery), have to respond to society's demands for safer procedures and to better cost management. As a result, the need for new approaches in surgical teaching has become apparent.

Also, training medical students in basic surgical maneuvers such as intestinal anastomosis could allow identification of those with special skills to be surgeons, as in the case of aviation [6].

Although the clinical impression, before the laparoscopic era, was that extramucosal one-layer running suture is as safe as interrupted suture in two layers, the need of simpler laparoscopic techniques has generalized the use of the former type and standardized learning [46, 47]. The difficulty associated with these laparoscopic anastomoses favored stapler use, with the consequent increase in financial costs, with no improvement in safety by comparison with a manual anastomosis performed by a skilled surgeon [1]. Nevertheless, other studies performed on ileo-colic anastomosis suggest higher leak rates in manual than in stapled anastomosis [34].

The appearance of assisted robotic surgery has increased the need for simplification of technical maneuvers, favoring the "manual" –through robotic arms- anastomosis, since the stapling devices are not incorporated into the robotic mechanisms.

Training Models

The first question that arises is: Which is the best model for teaching a basic technical skill such as intestinal anastomosis? Currently there are several options available: live animals, human bodies, inanimate models and virtual reality simulators. Although live animals and human bodies provide a more real anatomy and better tissue resistance, they are expensive. Technology improvement in virtual simulators has made them more attractive but they are also expensive and have limited synaptic feedback. Inanimate models are currently the best choice for anastomosis teaching. They are cheap and can be placed in any type of hospital or faculty, thus allowing easy access to staff surgeons, residents and medical students [5]. As a result they have become the central method for training in these skills.

Artificial Inanimate Models

These types of models have proven to be a good initial step in the learning of anastomosis technique, both open and laparoscopic, although their realism is poor.

Foam sponges: These were used with tubular shapes as the initial model both for manual and stapled intestinal anastomoses. They were cheap but with the disadvantages of lack of realism and are a difficult model to learn a proper technique [49].

Polyurethane foam: Later there appeared the polyurethane foams DASIE (Dog Abdominal Surrogate for Instructional Exercises) (DASIE International, Elora, Ontario, Canada), a model designed for developing some psychomotor skills needed for surgery. This model is used as an alternative to live animals to teach the sterile technique, instrument handling, suture procedures and abdominal surgery in general. It has an internal tube –the "intestine"- to practice different gastrointestinal sutures (anastomoses, ostomies). Its acceptance was assessed by means of a questionnaire answered by the staff of the Faculty where it was used. The results showed that DASIE worked well and was well accepted by trainees. It is considered an effective preparative method before practicing on live animals [50]. Other materials (collagen, polyester, expanded polytetrafluoroethylene (ePTFE): These materials, used for vascular prostheses, have also been applied as simulators, by using both ends as intestines which allow performing anastomoses of any type: end-to-end, end-to-side, side-to-side with the suture type designed by Lembert [51].

Flexible plastic materials: The original products consisted of a single layer flexible tubular structure. They let anastomosis be performed but this could not be "extramucosal". The trainee perception was that of stiffness higher than that of a human intestine. Later, these materials gained flexibility and manufacturers achieved a structure with two layers, very similar to the human intestine, and this allows performing a simulated extramucosal suture. The materials have also become more elastic and, therefore, more similar to the human intestine. As a result, training is more realistic both in open and laparoscopic surgery. Since these models are not expensive, they are included in the initial steps of the training programs for residents or medical students before inanimate models, live animals or human bodies [6].

Inanimate biological models: These models consist of animal viscus (usually pigs) used in experimental laboratories for training and then, sacrificed. Another possibility is to get them from pigs killed in industrial slaughterhouses. Quality and similarity with the human intestine depends on several factors:

a) Animal size: This is estimated by weight. To maximize the similarity with the human intestine diameter the animal weight must be over 150 kg. However, if the aim is the stomach or the colon, the weight ought not to exceed 30 kg.
b) Anatomic location of the viscus: Diameter increases from the proximal jejunum to the distal ileum, this being more similar to the human intestine.
c) Extraction time: Viscus obtained late after animal death –in case of dying because of hypovolemia during experimentation or training- lose much of the mucosa and the remaining layers get thinner after freezing. Therefore intestines obtained immediately after animal sacrifice are more convenient.
d) Handling and cleansing: The proper method to preserve viscus wall integrity is to wash it with water and glucose solution.
e) Freezing: The most real model is the fresh viscus, but in most cases it is necessary to freeze them for later use. This process must be performed quickly at low temperatures to preserve the viscus wall integrity. This is easier with stomachs but more difficult with intestine or colon. Defrosting must take a few hours and the viscus ought to be used immediately. Otherwise the mucosa loses its properties and the viscus becomes stiffer.

As a consequence of the freezing and defrosting processes, the perception during training is the tissues are more fragile and less elastic than human ones, leading to incomplete closure of the orifices produced by the needle (Figure 3). In addition, since the wall of most organs gets thinner, it is necessary to adjust better the size of the staplers, when used, to smaller calibers than in the live animal or the patient. In some viscus, such as the stomach, all the layers remain well preserved.

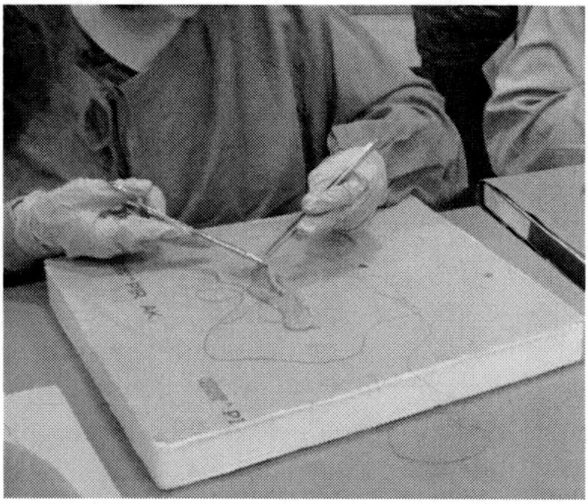

Figure 3.

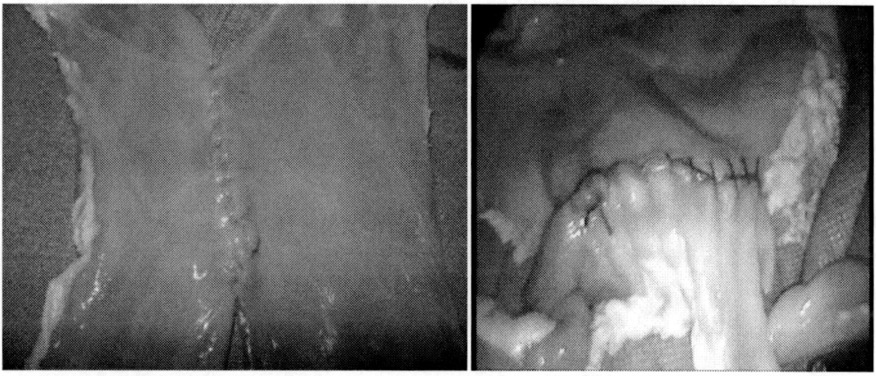

Figure 4. Pig viscus "*ex vivo*".

f) Anastomosis type: Small intestine is appropriate for manual or stapled side-to-side intestinal anastomosis, either open or laparoscopic, as well as for gastro-enteric anastomosis (Figure 4). However, it is less adequate for end-to-end anastomosis due to higher fragility and smaller size. The same situation occurs with the colon when performing a stapled end-to-end anastomosis [5, 52, 53].

Biological Models

These types increase the model complexity. They incorporate homeostatic phenomena characteristic of the biological elements. Their effects can be difficult to predict and control. Therefore, variability is a feature of biological models. As a result, experimental design is essential when dealing with these models.

The use of biological models, either animal or cadaveric, is associated with some ethical, moral and legal implications that it is necessary to bear in mind before planning training with these materials.

Animal Models

Live animal models are associated with the highest fidelity level by comparison with other models for training intestinal anastomosis performance. This is due to the possibility of operating on live viscus, with blood perfusion, not available in other models. Nevertheless, they cannot precisely represent human anatomy. Even the most similar and used, the porcine model, is flawed by important anatomic differences.

Live animal laboratories are expensive due to the need of anesthetic equipment, experienced personnel, and stabulation facilities. Also, several ethical considerations must have to be borne in mind when using live animals.

Pigs, rabbits and dogs have only one stomach and the small intestine is similar to the human one so they are useful for intestinal anastomosis training, either manual or stapled and irrespective of the approach, open or laparoscopic. For colo-rectal or ileo-colic anastomosis, pigs and dogs have more anatomical similarities to humans [54, 55], although ethical objections arise when dealing with dog use because of their affective proximity. The embryological development of the rabbit and the fact that it is a false ruminant make its large intestine wall stiffer and, therefore, a worse model. All those animals allow highly realistic training models. In addition it is possible to match their different sizes with those of newborns – rabbits -, children – small pigs – or adults - big pigs [56].

Since cadavers are seldom available and they are expensive, it has been shown that training on live animals is the best step before starting surgical practice on humans. As a result, the FLS (Fundamentals of Laparoscopic Surgery, a program offered by the American College of Surgeons and the SAGES-Society of American Gastrointestinal and Endoscopic Surgeons) includes training on pigs for residents and, for more advanced trainees, includes also practicing on cadavers [57].

Human Cadavers

The best option is to get fresh cadavers directly from pathology wards. This is the most realistic model but their continual availability to perform successive training sessions is limited [58]. An alternative is the fixation and preservation of cadavers by means of Walther Thiel's method [59] which allows body conservation in natural colors and texture. This is based on body immersion in a specific solution for a limited time. This method allows keeping the body out of the liquid and storing it in a closed container. If the body becomes too desiccated, it can be reintroduced in the solution to keep the tissues wet. This process leads to more convenient body handling and use. Also, since this process avoids formaldehyde use, there is no emission of irritant or damaging gases. The final result is a non-irritant and almost odorless body with high articular mobility, which retains tissue elasticity in a similar way to fresh bodies and, therefore, very adequate for training on invasive procedures.

A recent paper, which reviewed different studies concerning surgical training on human cadavers, suggested that technical skills acquired in low fidelity models (non-live models) could be as good as training on high fidelity models (cadavers), since the authors found that the learning process appears more important that the model itself [58]. This is especially true for procedures such as suture training which can be practiced on simulation models. These models, however, are probably not so advantageous when anatomical details and tissue fidelity play a more important role. This is the case of procedures such as viscus resection followed by stapled anastomosis (anterior low rectal resection) [60]. Another possible inconvenience to practice intestinal anastomosis is the higher stiffness of the intestinal wall and, as a result, more probabilities of tissue tear.

Nevertheless, the relationship between skills learned on cadavers and improvement in surgical results when operating directly on patients after objective assessment is not proven.

Anastakis describes cadaver models as the "gold standard for technical training". This can express a generalized opinion suggesting that it has to be the best model since it reproduces live human anatomy well. Cadaver models can be useful to allow trainees practicing procedures, with the possibility of making mistakes in a safe setting, before performing operations on patients [58].

Training Simulators

Physical simulators: These consist of containers to lodge *ex-vivo* viscus to perform anastomosis laparoscopically. They allow the placing of trocars to introduce the laparoscopic optical system and the instruments to perform different procedures. Physical simulators are very useful to do a wide variety of surgical procedures, without the need of using live animals (Figure 5). Also, they have been proven to be a good previous step before training on live animals, cadavers or patients [46].

Virtual simulators: Since the organism is very complex, it is necessary to simulate only the tissue biomechanical features, avoiding physiological processes such as bleeding. Even so, realistic simulation of the biomechanical behavior of human tissues is very difficult. The difficulty arises first from the scanty knowledge of the parameters which control tissue deformation. There is currently very little information concerning live tissue biomechanical features. This lack of information is due to technical troubles and ethical objections to measure these parameters on live tissues. As a result, the few available data come from dead pigs and human viscus. Since these viscuses do not have blood perfusion, the fast coagulation process inside and temperature difference significantly alter elasticity by comparison with live tissues. Therefore, these measures are hardly reliable.

Of note, the first virtual simulator used in anastomosis training was that of Boston Dynamics for vascular anastomosis, designed by Marc Raibert [61].

Simulator technology has developed fast since then. Concerning intestinal anastomosis simulators, however, only two current modules of Simbionix allow performing stapled anastomosis, for gastric by-pass [62] and another in the module of colo-rectal anastomosis. Hand suture is not possible in these simulators, which is a considerable limitation in training.

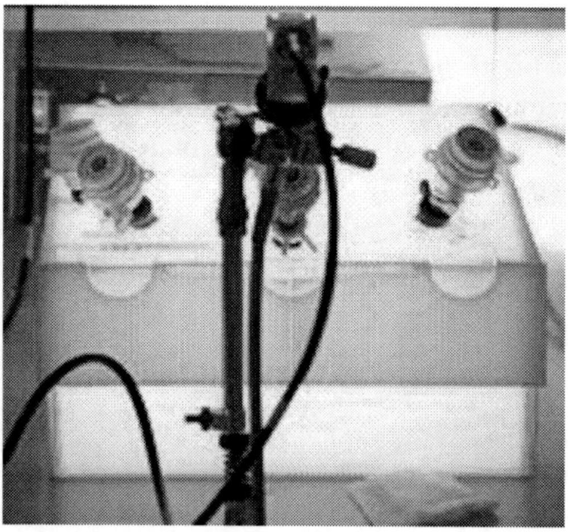

Figure 5. Physical simulator.

Training Models as a Mean to Assess Ability

Several scientific societies such as the American College of Surgeons (ACS), the Society of American Gastrointestinal and Endoscopic Surgeons (SAGES) with their training program FLS, the Royal College of Physicians and Surgeons of Canada, the Royal College of Surgeons of England and the Latin-American Federation of Surgery (FELAC) advise gastrointestinal anastomosis performance, both open and laparoscopic, for the resident curriculum to achieve basic technical ability in digestive surgery [63, 64, 65, 66, 67]. Moreover, the higher technical demands of laparoscopic surgery have forced many staff surgeons to train on anastomosis.

Several questions arise to know whether the above described models can fully develop surgical abilities.

a) Which training model could best help to achieve ability?

It has been shown that artificial models are a useful first step to adapt to the suture materials and staplers. Lauscher showed that intestinal anastomosis practicing in endotrainer with either a plastic digestive tube or animal viscus provides similar ability levels [68].

Virtual simulators cannot currently provide proper development of these techniques. Lewis suggests that the gastric by-pass module of the Simbionix virtual simulator only allows practicing the first steps of gastro-enteric stapled anastomosis [61].

Several authors have shown that inanimate biological models allow achieving technical ability and they state that this skill ought to be a previous step to direct training on live animals or human cadavers. Also, because of their low cost and high realism, the inanimate biological models ought to be used to decrease animal sacrifice. They allow the surgical techniques to be repeated many times, considering that the estimated training procedures necessary for proficiency are, at least, 8 anastomoses for open surgery, 4 in case of stapler use and 40 for manual laparoscopic anastomosis [5, 6, 46, 52]. Other authors describe, for the first steps of residents, ability achievement in terms of quality after doing 7 manual anastomoses, although the time spent is longer than the ideal [65].

In our opinion, the live biological models (experimental animals) and human body model allow achieving surgical abilities before the trainees operate directly on patients, and always after training on inanimate models in skill laboratories. Some authors have shown that practices on a small number of animals after using *ex-vivo* models provide the necessary ability [46, 55]. In the same way, the American College of Surgeons does not certify proficiency in these skills unless the trainee had practiced, first on live animals and, then, on cadavers. Anastakis found that assessments in cadaveric models are associated with higher scores than the live biological models [58].

b) How must training be developed before proficiency is reached?

Whatever ability is taught, it requires knowledge, training and communication: knowledge of the trainee about the procedure, previous training of the teacher and communication between them and with the environment during and after the process.

We think as does Peyton [69] that surgical training has several phases: demonstration, deconstruction, comprehension and yielding. The trainee has to pass from unconsciously incompetent to unconsciously competent.

The application of this theory to gastrointestinal anastomosis performance can be as follows: For the *"demonstration"* phase, videos illustrating the technique are used, as well as watching real procedures performed by expert surgeons, in a "no comment" way. The *deconstruction* phase allows defining the different steps of an anastomosis: extramucosal one-layer suture, angles performed according to Connell's technique and use of two threads tied in the middle of the posterior surface of the anastomosis; every thread goes to one side, performing a semi circumference with a running suture and, finally they are tied in the middle of the anterior surface. During the c*omprehension* phase, the mentor describes the previously detailed steps of the operation while doing the technique. Finally, in the *yielding* phase, the trainee "practices, practices and practices" until he or she gets an anastomosis of good enough quality and in adequate time. Throughout these phases and under expert supervision, the trainee goes from a setting of technical unawareness into another of technical knowledge. Meanwhile, the trainee assimilates the lessons, and the learning process passes from a conscious act into another automatic and unconscious one. At this moment, the learning process improves fast and is accelerated.

In our training laboratory for residents and young surgeons we have studied the learning process by doing intestinal anastomosis [5]. We found a decrease in the expected time and reduction of technical errors after training. We did however find a "plateau" after 70 hours of training, suggesting that practices offer little technical improvement beyond that time. We also observed (data not published) that the "automation" phase in case of manual laparoscopic anastomoses done in endotrainer is reached as of 40 procedures, although enough quality extramucosal suture and low leak rate had been achieved with 20. This means that the trainee has reached the conscious competent phase. Others have established as 50 manual anastomoses assisted by the Da Vinci robot the number necessary to equal in time and quality the anastomoses performed through an open approach [70, 71].

Since women have higher hand skill and men show better spatial coordination, possible learning differences have been proposed. However, studies have shown no difference in the final learning [6].

c) How can ability learning be assessed?

The ideal assessing system ought to be easy to use and to interpret, be accurate, reliable and acceptable. Objective systems of assessment by experts are the most reliable and useful, although only a few have the aforementioned features. Assessments based on video watching by experts need long time consumption and, therefore, are expensive and difficult to perform routinely.

Currently, assessment of technical skills depends on mentor qualification to a large degree.

Ability assessment based on objective models has several advantages. First, the abilities can be standardized in programs and, therefore, to evaluate specific skills. Second, objective assessment is possible but the scores could not correlate well with evaluation in the operating room. Actually, higher scores could induce the belief that the trainee is able to start practice on the patient before real proficiency has been reached.

To perform this, the Objective Structured Assessment of Technical Skills (OSATS) has been developed as a reliable method to assess abilities. This examination includes several items such as tissue handling, time to completion, knowledge and use of instruments, assistant managing, planning and development of operation and specific knowledge of the trained technique. A rating scale is built scoring each item from 0 to 5, according to a proper/improper performance criterion. Reznick [72] designed a type of OSATS examination to evaluate intestinal anastomoses in live animals.

The same authors as well as others [73, 74], use task check-lists to evaluate intestinal anastomosis addressing suture and knot quality as well as care of tissue handling. In our own experience, we assess anastomosis size, time to completion, suture quality (extramucosal stitches, eversion edge) and absence of leaks, as shown by means of hydrostatic tests [5]. This evaluation can be done by watching the videos recorded during training or by direct observation by the mentor.

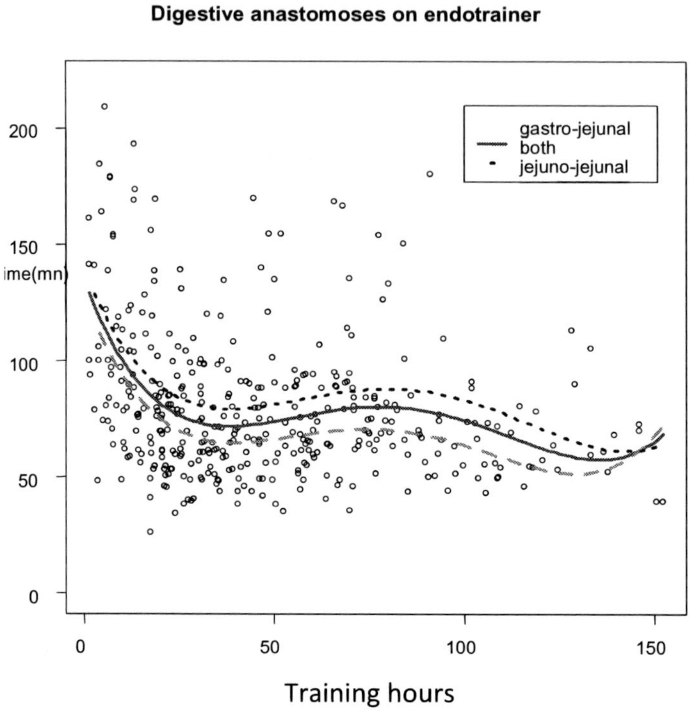

Figure 6. Correlation between time to anastomosis completion and hours of training.

The former allows evaluation by several experts and in different moments. The latter obliges the presence of evaluators in the training room and is usually limited to one or two people. The more structured and precise the check-lists are and the better experience is described, the higher the evaluation quality is. Quality is even higher when mentors have been properly trained in this methodology. The original OSATS were developed to be used as direct watching and then they were modified by authors such as Grantcharov to evaluate recorded procedures, where he found the rating scales were reliable enough to assess these tasks [75].

We did, in our training laboratory, direct structured watching by only one trained evaluator. After more than 5,000 anastomoses in a physical simulator, we found this assessing method is reliable to evaluate technical progression of surgical residents [5]. We think entero-enteric and gastro-enteric anastomoses are convenient techniques for laparoscopic training for several reasons. First, the time to completion can be measured and its decreasing can be correlated with time spent on training (Figure 6). Second, error rate decreases with training. However, learning does not improve over 70 hours' training, since beyond this period the time to completion and error rate decreasing is very low.

Assessment of Technical Skill Transfer from Simulation Models to the Patient in the Operating Room

Out of the reliable investigational setting, skill assessment in the operating room can be difficult. This is due to the possible variations in the operation designated to serve as evaluation, to the different academic standards and to the variation among the surgeons and residents in the way they perform the procedures. All of these lead to a lack of standardization and, therefore, to difficult evaluation.

Several questions arise before evaluating the transfer to the operating room. The first is whether endotrainer-based training is equivalent to the animal model.

We think as does Hamad [46] the surgical technique can be fully learned on a laparoscopic endotrainer, with repetition at least 40 times in a very standardized way. From our experience (data not published), a standardized technique such as the side-to-side gastro-enteric or entero-enteric anastomosis allows progression to the animal model when performed at least 40 times, with no improvement after further training.

Progression to live animal models demands adaptation to a less stable surgical field, more contaminated by fluids (blood, intestinal content), although the adaptation is usually fast. Hamad found in laparoscopic surgery a slight time increase in the performance of the different type of intestinal anastomoses (about 13 minutes), although without leaks or stenosis [46]. Others, such as Gonzalo Soto, found a mean time of 50 minutes with a failure rate of 3%, with no stenosis, after performance of 37 intestinal anastomoses [54].

When a bench model with open surgery instruments is used, the number of anastomoses and time required to equal expert results are lower, estimated as eight [6]. Staplers can help in the first steps of anastomoses.

In summary, we think the anastomoses ought to be trained in a standardized way, beginning on a bench or endotrainer model, and later pass to a live animal model. This skill can be achieved after doing the technique laparoscopically on both models about 50 times, and about 15 with an open approach. However, the transfer to patient is not yet established.

There are experiences with virtual simulators for training on laparoscopic cholecystectomy and laparoscopic gastric by-pass. Improvement in previous training to performing them directly on patients has been observed but, for the moment, virtual simulators for intestinal anastomosis exist only in the training field [61, 74].

Another question is whether the scoring systems (check-lists, OSATS) are able to discriminate, both in inanimate models and live models, the proficiency level achieved and whether this is enough to be transferred to the patient. Since there are no validated check-lists or OSATS for anastomoses, score systems of other procedures can be used, measuring time to completion and anastomosis quality. Most authors also include a pressure test to evaluate possible leaks.

Unfortunately, more factors influence anastomosis performance on patients, such as vascularization, end tension or patient-related factors (diabetes, corticosteroid intake). As a result, not only the technical skill, but also surgical clinical experience are determinant in succeeding when dealing with a patient.

References

[1] Bell RH Jr, Banker MB, Rhodes RS, Biester TW, Lewis FR. Graduate medical education in surgery in the United States. *Surg. Clin. North Am.,* 2007 Aug; 87(4): 811-23.

[2] Halsted WS. The training of the surgeon. *Bull. Johns. Hop. Hosp.,* 1904; 15:267-75.

[3] Cameron JL. William Stewart Halsted. Our surgical heritage. *Ann. Surg.,* 1997 May; 225(5): 445-58.

[4] Birkmeyer JD, Stukel TA, Siewers AE, Goodney PP, Wennberg DE, Lucas FL. Surgeon volume and operative mortality in the United States. *N. Eng. J. Med.,* 2003 Nov 27; 349 (22): 2117-27.

[5] Rodríguez-Sanjuán JC, Manuel-Palazuelos C, Fernández-Díez MJ, Gutiérrez JM, Alonso-Martín J, Redondo C, Herrera LA, Gómez-Fleitas M. Assessment of resident training in laparoscopic surgery based on a

digestive system anastomosis model in the laboratory. [Article in Spanish] *Cir. Esp.,* 2010 Jan; 87(1): 20-5.

[6] Masud D, Undre S, Darzi A. Using manual dexterity to predict the quality of the final product in the small bowel anastomosis after a period of training. *Am. J. Surg.,* 2012 Jun; 203(6): 776-81.

[7] Bann S, Darzi A. Selection of individuals for training in surgery. *Br. J. Surg.,* 2005; 190: 98 –102.

[8] Debas HT, Bass BL, Brennan MF, Flynn TC, Folse JR, Freischlag JA, et al. American Surgical Association Blue Ribbon Committee Report on Surgical Education: 2004. *Ann. Surg.,* 2005 Jan; 241(1):1-8.

[9] Scott DJ, Bergen PC, Laycock R, Tesfay ST, Valentine RJ, Euhus DM, et al. Laparoscopic training on bench models: better and more cost effective than operating room experience? *J. Am. Coll. Surg.,* 2000;191: 272-83.

[10] Seymour NE, Gallagher AG, Roman SA, O'Brien MK, Bansal VK, Andersen DK, et al. Virtual reality training improves operating room performance: results of a randomized, double-blinded study. *Ann. Surg.,* 2002; 236:458-63.

[11] Fried GM, Feldman LS, Vassiliou MC, Fraser SA, Stanbridge D, Ghitulescu G, et al. Proving the value of simulation in laparoscopic surgery. *Ann. Surg.,* 2004; 240:518-25.

[12] Sroka G, Feldman LS, Vassiliou MC, Kaneva PA, Fayez R, Fried GM. Fundamentals of laparoscopic surgery simulator training to proficiency improves laparoscopic performance in the operating room---a randomized controlled trial. *Am. J. Surg.,* 2010; 199:115-20.

[13] Tan SS, Sarker SK. Simulation in surgery: a review. *Scott. Med. J.,* 2011 May;56(2):104-9.

[14] Sutherland LM, Middleton PF, Anthony A, Hamdorf J, Cregan P, Scott D, Maddern GJ. Surgical simulation: a systematic review. *Ann. Surg.,* 2006 Mar; 243 (3): 291-300.

[15] Chen C. The art of bowel anastomosis. *Scand. J. Surg.,* 2012;101(4):238-40.

[16] Bernard CL, Huette C. Procédé de Lembert. In Précis iconographique de médecine opératoire et d'anatomie chirurgicale. Paris: *Méquignon-*Marvis, 1855, p. 257, pl. 59 p. 260-261 (495 p.).

[17] Lembert A: Memoire sur l'enterorraphie avec description d'un precede nouveau pour pratiquer cette operation chirurgicale. *Rep. Gen. D'Anat. Physiol. Pathol. Clin. Chir.,* 1826;2:100–107.

[18] Halsted WS: Circular structure of the intestine: an experimental study. *Am. J. Med. Sci.,* 1887; 94:436–461.

[19] Murphy JB. Cholecysto-intestinal, gastrointestinal, enterointestinal anastomosis and approximation without sutures. *Med. Rec.,* 1892; 42:665-676.

[20] Forde KA, McLarty AJ, Tsai J, Ghalili K, Delany HM. Murphy's button revisited: Clinical experience with the biofragmentable anastomotic ring. *Ann. Surg.,* 1993; 217:78–81.

[21] Ravitch MM, Brown IW, Daviglus GF: Experimental and clinical use of the Soviet Bronchus Stapling Instruments. *Surgery,* 1959; 46:1-97.

[22] Hesp FL, Hendriks T, Lubbers EJ, deBoer HH. Wound healing in the intestinal wall. A comparison between experimental ileal and colonic anastomoses. *Dis. Colon. Rectum.,* 1984 Feb; 27(2): 99-104.

[23] Wise L, McAlister W, Stein T, Schuck P. Studies on the healing of anastomoses of small and large intestines. *Surg. Gynecol. Obstet.,* 1975 Aug;141(2):190-194.

[24] Matthiessen P, Hallböök O, Rutegård J, Simert G, Sjödahl R. Defunctioning stoma reduces symptomatic anastomotic leakage after low anterior resection of the rectum for cancer: a randomized multicentre trial. *Ann. Surg.,* 2007 Aug;246(2):207-214.

[25] Schrock TR, Deveney CW, Dunphy JE. Factors contributing to leakage of colonic anastomoses. *Ann. Surg.,* 1973; 177(5):513-518.

[26] Paterson-Brown S, Beck DE, Whitlow CB. A Companion to Specialist Surgical Practice: Core Topics in General and Emergency Surgery. 4th ed. Philadelphia: *Elsevier. Saunders,* 2009: 167-192.

[27] Sørensen LT, Jørgensen T, Kirkeby LT, Skovdal J, Vennits B, Wille-Jørgensen P. Smoking and alcohol abuse are major risk factors for anastomotic leakage in colorectal surgery. *Br. J. Surg.,* 1999; 86(7):927-931.

[28] Witte MB, Barbul A: repair of full-thickness bowel injury. *Crit. Care. Med.,* 2003;31:S 538–546.

[29] Goligher J, McAdam W. A controlled trial of inverting versus everting intestinal suture in clinical large bowel surgery. *Br. J. Surg.,* 1970; 57:817.

[30] Miettinen RP, Laitinen ST, Mäkelä JT, Pääkkönen ME. Bowel preparation with oral polyethylene glycol electrolyte solution vs. no preparation in elective open colorectal surgery: prospective, randomized study. *Dis. Colon. Rectum.,* 2000; 43 (5); 669-675.

[31] Bucher P, Gervaz P, Morel P: Should preoperative mechanical bowel preparation be abandoned? *Ann. Surg.,* 2007; 245(4): 662.
[32] Goulder F. Bowel anastomoses: The theory, the practice and the evidence baseWorld *J. Gastrointest. Surg.,* 2012 September 27; 4(9): 208-213.
[33] Docherty JG, McGregor JR, Akyol AM, Murray GD, Galloway DJ. Comparison of manually constructed and stapled anastomoses in colorectal surgery. West of Scotland and Highland Anastomosis Study Group. *Ann. Surg.,* 1995 Feb; 221(2): 176-184.
[34] Choy PY, Bissett IP, Docherty JG, Parry BR, Merrie AE. Stapled versus handsewn methods for ileocolic anastomoses. *Cochrane Database Syst. Rev.,* 2007: CD004320.
[35] Simillis C, Purkayastha S, Yamamoto T, Strong SA, Darzi AW, Tekkis PP. A meta-analysis comparing conventional end-to-end anastomosis vs. other anastomotic configurations after resection in Crohn's disease. *Dis. Colon. Rectum.,* 2007 Oct; 50(10): 1674-1687.
[36] McLeod RS, Wolff BG, Ross S, Parkes R, McKenzie M. Recurrence of Crohn's disease after ileocolic resection is not affected by anastomotic type: results of a multicenter, randomized, controlled trial. *Dis. Colon. Rectum.,* 2009; 52: 919-927.
[37] Taflampas P, Christodoulakis M, Tsiftsis DD. Anastomotic leakage after low anterior resection for rectal cancer: facts, obscurity, and fiction. *Surg. Today,* 2009; 39(3):183-188.
[38] Brundage SI, Jurkovich GJ, Grossman DC, Tong WC, Mack CD, Maier RV. Stapled versus sutured gastrointestinal anastomoses in the trauma patient. *J. Trauma.,* 1999; 47: 500-507; discussion 500-507.
[39] Brundage SI, Jurkovich GJ, Hoyt DB, Patel NY, Ross SE, Marburger R, Stoner M, Ivatury RR, Ku J, Rutherford EJ, Maier RV. Stapled versus sutured gastrointestinal anastomoses in the trauma patient: a multicenter trial. *J. Trauma,* 2001; 51: 1054-1061.
[40] Jyoti Shah, Yaron Munz, Joanne Manson, Krishna Moorthy, Ara Darzi. Objective Assessment of Small Bowel Anastomosis Skill in Trainee General Surgeons and Urologists. *World J. Surg.,* (2006) 30: 248–251.
[41] Jörn Gröne, Jörg-Peter Ritz, Andrea Stroux, Kai S. Lehmann, Johannes C. Lauscher. Measurable learning effects after a 1-week skills course in digestive surgery. *Int. J. Colorectal. Dis.,* (2010) 25:1133–1139.
[42] Slawomir J. Marecik, Vivek Chaudhry, Azam Jan, Russell K. Pearl, John J. Park, Leela M. Prasad. A comparison of robotic, laparoscopic,

and hand-sewn intestinal sutured anastomoses performed by residents. *The American Journal of Surgery,* 193 (2007) 349–355.

[43] Goligher JC, Lee PW, Simpkins KC, Lintott DJ. A controlled comparison one- and two-layer techniques of suture for high and low colorectal anastomoses. *Br. J. Surg.,* 1977; 64: 609-614.

[44] Maurya SD, Gupta HC, Tewari A, Khan SS, Sharma BD. Double layer versus single layer intestinal anastomosis: a clinical trial. *Int. Surg.,* 1984; 69:339-340.

[45] Shikata S, Yamagishi H, Taji Y, Shimada T, Noguchi Y. Single- versus two- layer intestinal anastomosis: a meta-analysis of randomized controlled trials. *BMC Surg.,* 2006; 6:2.

[46] Hamad MA, Mentges B, Buess G. Laparoscopic sutured anastomosis of the bowel; Technique and learning curve. *Surg. Endosc.,* 2003; 17: 1840-1844.

[47] Max E, Sweeney WB, Bailey HR, Oommen SC, Butts DR, Smith KW, Zamora LF, Skakun GB. Results of 1000 single-layer continuous polypropylene intestinal anastomoses. *Am. J. Surg.,* 1991; 162:461– 467.

[48] Mohr Z, Willis S. Intestinal anastomoses and techniques in the lower gastrointestinal tract. *Chirurg,* 2011;82:34-40.

[49] Ramos-Salgado F, Quintero-Becerra J, Hernández-Toriz N. Modelo para entrenamiento de cirugía laparoscópica urológica. *Rev. Mex. Urol.,* 2010; 70:31-35.

[50] Holmberg D.L, Cockshutt JR, Basher A. Use of a dog abdominal surrogate for teaching surgery. *J. Vet. Med. Educ.,* 1993; 20:107-111.

[51] Molina Martínez JL, Silveira Prado E, et al. Simulators and experimental models for the development of surgical skills on the Health Sciences teaching–learning process REDVET Rev. electrón. vet. http://www.veterinaria.org/revistas/redvet 2012 Volumen 13, Nº 6.

[52] Vick L, Kenneth D. Borman K, and Salameh JR. Face, Content, and Construct Validities of Inanimate Intestinal Anastomoses Simulation. *Journal of Surgical Education,* 2007; 64: 365-368.

[53] Munksdorf M, Fischer A, Hoffmann J. Experiences with surgical training in anastomosis technics using porcine gut. *Ugeskr. Laeger.,* 1990;152:2575-6.

[54] Gonzalo Soto D, George Pinedo M, Demian Fullerton M, Francisca León G, Francisco Lopez K. Hand-sewn anastomosis in laparoscopic colon surgery. An experimental model. *Rev. Chilena de Cirugía,* 2005; 57: 149-154.

[55] Jardel N, Hidalgo A, Leperlier D, Manassero M, Gomes A, Bedu AS, Moissonnier P, Fayolle P, Begon D, Riquois E, Viateau V. One Stage Functional End-to-End Stapled Intestinal Anastomosis and Resection Performed by Non expert Surgeons for the Treatment of Small Intestinal Obstruction in 30 Dogs. *Veterinary Surgery,* 2011; 40: 216–222.

[56] Kirlum HJ, Heinrich M, Till H: The rabbit model serves as a valuable operative experience and helps to establish new techniques for abdominal and thoracic endosurgery. *Pediatr. Surg. Int.,* 2005; 21: 91-93.

[57] Palter V, and Grantcharov T. Development and validation of a Comprehensive Curriculum to Teach an Advanced Minimally Invasive Procedure. A Randomized Controlled Trial. *Ann. Surg.,* 2012; 256:25-32.

[58] Anastakis DJ, Regehr G, Reznick RK, et al. Assessment of technical skills transfer from the bench training model to the human model. *Am. J. Surg.,* 1999;177:167–170.

[59] Thiel, W. Die Konservierung ganzer Leichen in natürlichen Farben. *Ann. Anat.,* 1992; 174: 185-195.

[60] Gilbody J, Prasthofer AW, Ho K, Costa ML. The use and effectiveness of cadaveric workshops in higher surgical training: a systematic review. *Ann. R. Coll. Surg. Engl.,* 2011;93:347-52.

[61] Satava R, Jones S. Preparación de cirujanos para el siglo XXI. Consecuencias de los avances tecnológicos. Cirugía muy poco invasora parte I. *Surg. Clin. N. Am.,* 2000; 4:1417-1429.

[62] Lewis T, Aggarwal R, Kwasnicki R, Rajaretnam N, Moorthy K, Ahmed A, Darzi A. Can virtual reality simulation be used for advanced bariatric surgical training? *Surgery,* 2012;151:779-84.

[63] Mittal MK, Dumon KR, Edelson PK, Acero NM, Hashimoto D, Danzer E, Selvan B, Resnick AS, Morris JB, Williams NN. Successful Implementation of the American College of Surgeons/Association of Program Directors in Surgery Surgical Skills Curriculum via a 4-Week Consecutive Simulation Rotation. *Simul. Healthc.,* 2012; 7:147-54.

[64] Vassiliou M, Dunkin BJ, Marks JM, MDc, Fried G M., FLS and FES: Comprehensive Models of Training and Assessment. *Surg. Clin. N. Am.,* 2010; 90: 535–558.

[65] Chan B, Martel G, Poulin E, Mamazza J, Boushey R. Resident training in minimally invasive surgery: a survey of Canadian department and division chairs. *Surg. Endosc.,* 2010; 24:499–503

[66] Olson T, Becker Y, McDonald R, Gould J. A Simulation-Based Curriculum Can Be Used to Teach Open Intestinal Anastomosis. *Journal of Surgical Research,* 2012; 172, 53–58.

[67] A. Jensen. A. Andrew. Laboratory based instruction for skin closure and bowel ansstomosis for surgical residents. *Arch. Surg.,* 2008; 143:852-859.

[68] Lauscher JC, Ritz JP, Stroux A, Buhr HJ, Gro¨ne, J. A New Surgical Trainer (BOPT) Improves Skill Transfer for Anastomotic Techniques in Gastrointestinal Surgery into the Operating Room: A Prospective Randomized Trial. *World J. Surg.,* 2010; 34: 2017– 2025.

[69] Peyton JWR. The learning cycle. In: Peyton JWR, editor. Teaching and learning in medical practice. Rickmansworth, UK: Manticore Europe Limited, 1998: 13-19.

[70] Pearl RK, Park J, Prasad L. A comparison of robotic, laparoscopic, and hand-sewn intestinal sutured anastomoses performed by residents. *The American Journal of Surgery,* 2007;193: 349–355.

[71] Marecik SJ, Prasad L, Park J, Jan A, Chaudhry V. Evaluation of midlevel and upper-level residents performing their first robotic-sutured intestinal anastomosis. *American Journal of Surgery,* 2008;195: 333–338.

[72] Martin JA, Regehr G, Reznick R et al. Objective structured assessment of technical skill (OSATS) for surgical residents. *Br. J. Surg.,* 1997; 84: 273 – 278.

[73] Reznick R, Regehr G, MacRae H et al. Testing technical skill via an innovative ''bench station'' examination. *Am. J. Surg.,* 1997; 173:226–230.

[74] Chipman JG, Schmitz C. Using Objective Structured Assessment of Technical Skills to Evaluate a Basic Skills Simulation Curriculum for First-Year Surgical Residents. *J. Am. Coll Surg.,* 2009; 209: 364-370.

[75] Kundhal PS, Grantcharov TP. Psychomotor performance measured in a virtual environment correlates with technical skills in the operating room. *Surg. Endosc.,* 2009; 23:645–649.

In: Anastomoses ISBN: 978-1-62618-657-6
Editors: F. King, McKineley A. Malloy © 2013 Nova Science Publishers, Inc.

Chapter III

Invaginating Colonic Anastomosis

Aly Saber*
Port-Fouad General Hospital, Department of general surgery
Port-Fouad, Port-Said, Egypt

1. Historical Background

The earliest reports of surgical suture date back to 3000 BC in ancient Egypt, and the oldest known suture is in a mummy from 1100 BC. The ancient Egyptians and Babylonians and the later Greeks and Romans used the intestines of herbivorous animals for much the same purposes. Detailed records of sigmoid volvulus were found in the Egyptian Papyrus Ebers and in ancient Greek and Roman writings. The ancient Egyptian Ebers papyrus describes the natural history of sigmoid volvulus as either reducing spontaneously, or the sigmoid colon being 'rotted'. Written in 500 BCE, the detailed description of a wound suture and the suture materials used in it is by the Indian sage and physician Sushruta.

Early in the first century AD, Celsus recorded attempts to suture the intestine but and Abulkasem in 87 AD, recommended using the jaws of large ants to unite intestinal wounds and referred to catgut made from the intestines

* E-mail: Alysaber54@gmail.com.

of sheep as suture material. Other ancient surgical methods involved the use of a few large-diameter sutures; use of bone, trachea, or wood stents; or attempt to invaginate the cut ends of intestine. The oldest reported intestinal suturing technique is the Glover's suture that was a simple continuous stitch in which the ends, instead of being tied, were left long and pulled externally through the abdominal wound.

Current principles of intestinal surgery originated in the early 19th century. In 1812, Travers first reported that the entire circumference of the divided intestine needed to be in contact to heal properly. Travers used a small; round sewing needle to place multiple full-thickness silk sutures and knotted the sutures. He reported successful healing of intestinal anastomoses in dogs with his mucosal appositional and everting technique. In 1826, Lembert, the founder of modern intestinal surgery, reported that serosa-to-serosa contact of the divided intestine, achieved by inverting suture patterns, was necessary for intestinal healing and became a fundamental principle of intestinal surgery. In 1883, Czerny modified Lembert's technique into a two-layer, inverting anastomosis, which became widely used in the 20th century. In 1887, Halsted reported the importance of the submucosal layer in suturing gut wounds using a single-layer closure. In 1892, Connell introduced a single-layer, continuous inverting suture pattern with the advantages of reduction of the number of knots left in the wound and operative time.

In 1892 also, Murphy described the use of an inter-locking metallic button designed to create a sutureless, inverting, end-to-end intestinal anastomosis and the button finally would pass with the feces. Nevertheless, Murphy's button was largely replaced by hand-sewn intestinal anastomosis techniques in human patients by the 1920s. By the beginning of the 20th century, about 250 methods for intestinal suturing had been described with these principles: (1) opposing the serosal surfaces of the intestine around the full circumference using an inverting suture technique, (2) including the tough submucosa in the suture bites,(3) using aseptic surgical technique, (5)maintaining adequate blood supply to tissue, and (6) avoiding tension on the anastomosis.

Information on surgical treatment of intestinal diseases in the small animal veterinary literature is generally lacking before the1940s. The first edition of Canine Surgery was published in 1939. In a 1941 small animal surgery textbook, McCann stated that the prognosis is always grave for enterorrhaphy in the dog. The textbook described use of an inverting Lembert pattern to perform end-to-end small intestinal anastomosis and mentioned various mechanical devices, such as the Murphy button, that require no sutures. McCunn admitted that, in his experience with enterorrhaphy, the results were not good, although there had been some successes. In 1951, Gambee described a single-layer, inverting technique for intestinal anastomosis. He reported good results with the technique in comparison of double-layer closure in the GI tract, which was widely used in human surgery. The first challenges to Lembert's principles of inversion and serosal contact also appeared in the 1950s. The earliest descriptions of everting intestinal anastomoses in the veterinary literature appeared in the 1960s. In 1968, Ott and colleagues compared single layer, inverting anastomosis with everting anastomosis in the small intestine of dogs. They concluded that the everting technique was stronger and was associated with less compromise of the lumen diameter and fewer complications.

The first report of simple interrupted approximating anastomosis has become the technique of choice for end-to-end anastomosis in small animal surgery appeared in1970 when Bennett and Zydeck and in 1973, DeHoff and co- workers compared single-layer everting, inverting, and approximating end-to-end jejunal anastomoses in dogs and puppies. In 1976, Reinerts compared three patterns for equine jejunal anastomosis: a modified Gambee appositional suture, a simple interrupted everting suture, and a double-row inverting suture. In 1981, Ellison reviewed techniques for end-to-end intestinal anastomosis in dogs and pointed out the difficulty in avoiding some degree of mucosal eversion with proper surgical technique and stated that any anastomotic suture pattern could be used successfully in the canine intestine. In 1982, Ellison and colleagues reported that the needle passage should to exclude the mucosa in an attempt to minimize eversion. In 1982, Bellenger was the first to report results of experimental appositional anastomosis and single-layer inverting of the jejunum in cats. Recently, Weisman and colleagues reported that modified simple continuous pattern for closure of intestinal incisions is an acceptable alternative to the simple interrupted pattern in dogs and cats. Reported advantages of a simple continuous enteric closure include surgical speed, decreased tissue handling, improved apposition of intestinal layers, and a low rate of clinical complications. Simple continuous approximating anastomosis has been shown experimentally to achieve better continuity of the histologic intestinal layers than do simple interrupted approximating techniques.

The current automated stapling instruments for intestinal anastomosis originated in the former Soviet Union after World War II. These stapling devices were first tested in the United States in the 1960s and became widely accepted for use in human surgical patients in the 1970s. Hess and coworkers published the first veterinary study that compared mechanically stapled with hand-sewn small intestinal anastomoses. Although the outcomes of the two techniques were similar, the mechanical staples were applied more consistently and required less surgical time than did the sutures. Stoloff and colleagues and in 1991, Ullman and colleagues in separate works, compared stapled and hand-sewn colonic anastomoses in dogs. They reported less tissue reaction, improved healing, and fewer adhesions with the inverted stapled anastomosis.

A biofragmentable ring composed of polyglycolic acid for intestinal anastomosis has been experimentally tested in dogs and cats and has been used clinically in humans that is similar to the Murphy button but breaks down approximately 12 days after implantation and eventually pass with the feces. Experimental data show that colonic anastomoses achieved with a biofragmentable ring have higher initial bursting strength and similar healing patterns compared with sutured and stapled anastomoses. Clinical application of the biofragmentable anastomosis ring has not been reported in the veterinary literature.

2. Techniques of Colonic Anastomosis

2.1. Principles of Successful Intestinal Anastomosis

Intestinal anastomosis is one of the most commonly performed surgical procedures, especially in the emergency setting, and is also commonly performed in the elective setting when resections are carried out for benign or malignant lesions of the gastrointestinal tract. Proper surgical technique and adherence to the following fundamental principles are imperative to ensure successful outcome after intestinal anastomosis. The first principle of proper technique for intestinal anastomoses is adequate exposure as the intestine should be mobilized sufficiently for proper anastomosis. Sufficient serosa must be exposed so that the seromuscular sutures or staples can be placed directly in the serosa without traversing the mesentery. The second principle is to maintain a good blood supply to the severed ends of the bowel. The blood supply may be compromised by construction of an anastomosis under tension, excessive dissection or mobilization of the bowel, excessive use of the electrocautery, and tying of the sutures so tight that the intervening tissue is strangulated. The third principle involves prevention of local spillage of enteric contents. The best way of preventing spills is to operate on prepared bowel Local spills and local sepsis have an adverse effect on the healing anastomosis, and it is for this reason that noncrushing occlusion clamps, in addition to an adequate bowel preparation, are advisable. The fourth principle is an accurate apposition of serosa to serosa of the two segments of bowel to be anastomosed. The anastomosis should be watertight and performed without tension. The bowel must be handled gently with the use of noncrushing forceps. The fifth principle is absence of tension and distal obstruction with gentle and meticulous tissue handling technique. The final principle involves realignment of the mesentery of the two segments of bowel to be joined with good approximation of well vascularized cut ends of the bowel. These should be parallel to each other and ensure that there is no twist on completion of the anastomosis.

2.2. Suture Materials

Successful wound healing depends on an appropriate tensile strength provided by the suture materials and a microenvironment in which the repaired tissues are likely to attach and grow. Choice of suture materials includes an absorbable versus nonabsorbable material, monofilament versus polyfilament. Nonabsorbable sutures can retain their tensile strength for one year or longer, whereas the half-lives of tensile strength for absorbable sutures vary from one to several weeks. Suture materials are required in practically every surgical operation and most researchers think that some of the complications following surgery may be directly attributable to the suture material itself. The observations indicate that anastomotic suture support is of minor or no importance one to two weeks after the procedure. There are four important properties common to all suture materials: the intensity of the inflammatory response which the particular material evokes in the tissues; the behavior of the material in the presence of infection; its durability; and its handling ability. The degree of tissue reaction caused by the sutures has two important consequences. Firstly, an excessive tissue reaction will lead to impairment of the strength of the tissues and this decreases the holding power of the stitches, which consequently tend to leak. Accordingly, materials which cause the least tissue reaction generally produce the strongest closure. Secondly, there is some evidence that infection is more likely to occur in wounds sutured with materials causing excessive tissue reaction. Sutures act as foreign bodies in the anastomosis, producing inflammation which persists for two or three weeks. Inflammation seems to delay the healing of an intestinal anastomosis and the ideal suture provokes a minimal inflammatory response. Thus modern, synthetic, absorbable suture materials can be used safely for intestinal anastomosis. Absorption of the suture material eliminates the foreign body residue seen with nonabsorbable sutures that induces a strong tissue reaction. Absorbable sutures are made of natural materials which are broken down in tissue after a short period of time, ranging from days to few weeks. In most cases, three weeks is sufficient for the wound to close firmly. The suture is not needed any more, and the fact that it disappears is an advantage, as there is no foreign material left inside the body and no need for the patient to have the sutures removed. Absorbable sutures were originally made of the intestines of sheep, the so called catgut. Today, gut sutures are made of specially prepared beef and sheep intestine, and may be untreated (plain gut), tanned with chromium salts to increase their persistence in the body (chromic gut), or heat-treated to give more rapid absorption (fast gut). However, the majority of absorbable sutures are now made of synthetic polymer fibres, which may be braided or monofilament; these offer numerous advantages over gut sutures, notably ease of handling, low cost, low tissue reaction, consistent performance and guaranteed non-toxicity.

Non absorbable sutures are made of materials which are not metabolized by the body, and are used therefore either on skin wound closure, where the sutures can be removed after a few weeks, or in some inner tissues in which absorbable sutures are not adequate. This is the case, for example, in the heart and in blood vessels, whose rhythmic movement requires a suture which stays longer than three weeks, to give the wound enough time to close. Other organs, like the bladder, contain fluids which make absorbable sutures disappear in only a few days, too early for the wound to heal. There are several materials used for non absorbable sutures. The most common is a natural fibre, silk, which undergoes a special manufacturing process to make it adequate for its use in surgery. Other non-absorbable sutures are made of artificial fibres, like polypropylene, polyester or nylon; these may or may not have coatings to enhance their performance characteristics. Finally, stainless steel wires are commonly used in orthopaedic surgery and for sternal closure in cardiac surgery.

2.3. Anastomotic Pattern

There are many types of intestinal anastomotic patterns available in human and veterinary practices. However, there is no universal agreement about the best technique for gastrointestinal anastomosis (GIA). Predicted fear of increased postoperative complications secondary to the anastomotic failure has resulted in a diversity of techniques. The type of gastrointestinal anastomotic construction is usually left to the choice of the surgeon, according to his experience and preference for hand- sewn or stapled sutures. Anastomotic patterns are typically categorized as sutured, stapling and sutureless anastomosis. The sutured anastomosis may be continuous or interrupted, single layer or double layers and inverting, appositional, or everting. The two-layer anastomosis using interrupted silk sutures for an outer inverted seromuscular layer and a running absorbable suture for a transmural inner layer has been standard for most surgical situations. Some recent reports have described single-layer continuous anastomosis using monofilament sutures as requiring less time and cost than any other method, without incurring any added risk of leakage. Many surgeons probably now use single-layer suturing due to reductions in ischemia, tissue necrosis or narrowing of the lumen compared to the two-layer method. The interrupted serosubmucosal suture was considered as the "gold standard" for intestinal anastomosis with many advantages as: accurate tissue apposition, incorporates submucosa, minimizes damage to submucosal vascular plexus, lesser tissue strangulation, appropriate for both upper and lower GI tract anastomosis and appropriate for both accessible and inaccessible sites.

Stapling technology was pioneered in the early part of this century and subsequently modified. Russian initiatives led to development of the original circular stapling instrument and further progress has resulted in instruments that are widely available, reliable and totally disposable. Mechanical failure is now rare and malfunction is generally due to operator error. Complications related to the stapling technique are uncommon, although anastomotic stricture may be more frequent than when hand- sewn anastomosis is performed. A stapling instrument facilitates and may expedite a surgical procedure but it is an adjunct to, and not a substitute for, meticulous surgical technique. The safety, efficacy, and technique of stapled gastrointestinal tract anastomosis in adults have been extensively documented since 1978. Recently, a single-stapled technique was performed instead of the conventional double-stapled technique in laparoscopic low anterior resection for anastomosis, by placement of intracorporeal purse-string sutures on the distal rectum with transanal specimen extraction. The stapler has many advantages: a better blood supply, less tissue manipulation, minimal edema, uniformity of sutures, easy lumen calibration and short operative times.

The concept of a sutureless intestinal anastomosis has been attractive to surgeons for many years. Beginning in the early 19th century, surgical investigators have designed ingenious but often complicated devices to achieve end-to-end intestinal anastomosis. Sutureless intestinal anastomoses can be achieved either by compression, where two inverted rings of bowel are compressed by a hollow circular device that subsequently sloughs away and is passed through the anus, or by the use of tissue glues or laser welding. Compression devices used clinically with success are the Valtrac biofragmentable anastomotic ring, the polypropylene rings described by Rosati and the AKA guns. Glued anastomoses have only been used in animals and seem to be unsafe. However, laser-welded intestinal anastomoses appear highly promising in experimental studies and further development of this technique is warranted.

3. Anastomotic Line Protection

The relative high incidence of anastomotic leakage after colorectal surgery, with its major consequences for morbidity and mortality, remain of great concern. Accordingly, researchers tried to use many techniques and devices to protect the anastomotic site.

3.1. External Coating

External coating of colonic anastomoses has been proposed as a means to lower the rate of anastomotic complication. A number of external anastomosis reinforcements have been tested, including peritoneal graft, omental graft, dura mater, and meshes. Omentum is the tissue most often used for anastomosis reinforcement. Several studies suggested that omental reinforcement prevents anastomosis leakage, whereas others found that this approach caused an increased risk of infection associated with pedicular necrosis or late intestinal obstruction. Both human dura mater and free peritoneal graft reinforcement showed reduced anastomosis healing that could be attributed to avascularity of grafts and to aggravated adhesions between anastomosis and intra-abdominal organs and consequently led to decreased anastomosis healing. Non-absorbable meshes reinforce anastomoses permanently, however, may increase the risk of peritoneal adhesion, anastomotic stenosis, and colon perforation, in the long term. In experimental animals, fibrin sealant was used and showed increased bursting pressure and rupture strength of colonic anastomoses. Hyaluronic acid-carboxymethylcellulose also was used in rats to protect the anastomotic lines and further studies have to be performed. Accordingly, the external coating of colonic anastomoses has yet failed to show convincing results.

3.2. Luminal Devices

Intra-luminal colonic devices are used in both animal studies and human aiming to prevent the faecal load from contacting the anastomotic site, thereby preventing leakage of faeces into the peritoneal cavity when the walls of the anastomosis have become dehiscent. When the faecal stream is bypassed from contacting the bowel mucosa, a gap in the anastomosis will not lead to extravasation of intra-luminal content.

3.2.1. Animal Studies

Coloshield

In the 1980's, Ravo and Ger developed an intraluminal colonic tube to prevent anastomotic leakage. The proximal end of the tube is fixed to the proximal bowel loop using polyglycolic acid sutures. Studies on dogs were performed using different tubes varying in width and length, material (latex, silicone, rubber), and suture technique.

The colon tube placement was found to be a safe, uncomplicated procedure and none of the dogs developed leak. All tubes were allowed to be expelled naturally together with the faecal stream.

Silicone Prosthesis

The intracolonic silicone prosthesis in protecting the anastomosis in dogs was used since 1992.

Soft Latex Tube

Intraluminal colonic soft latex tubes were studied by Ross in a rat model and the results suggested that the intraluminal tubes have a survival advantage compared to controls without tubes.

Polyflex Self-Expandable Covered Plastic Stent

In 2008 Tsereteli et al. performed their study in pigs comparing the incidence of anastomotic leak after open rectosigmoid resection with or without a Polyflex self-expandable covered plastic stent. The stent was placed over a guide wire with use of a flexible colonoscope and deployed under fluorescence control.

This experiment demonstrated a significant beneficial effect of the stent as a breakthrough solution for the complicated colorectal anastomosis, avoiding the necessity of a stoma during the healing process.

3.2.2. Human Studies

Coloshield

The development of the intraluminal tube led to the final version of the Coloshield to be a soft, pliable tube like a surgical glove. This intraluminal protective device, developed by Ravo, was first used in humans in 1984. Indications for use include perforated diverticulitis, colonic obstruction, volvulus, carcinoma, and fistula. Several non-randomized studies were performed in patients undergoing colon surgery with the Coloshield. In 1991, Ravo described a method of inserting the Coloshield in the proximal colon after completion of the anastomosis by performing a longitudinal colostomy on the antimesenteric border of the afferent loop, proximal to the anastomosis. Ravo and Ger pioneered the use of intracolonic stents, testing different materials (silicone, rubber, and latex) before developing and, finally, filing the patent of the latex Coloshield. Despite its promise, the Coloshield has not been widely accepted.

Condom

In 1994, Yoon et al. and in 1995, Ruiz et al. used a condom instead of a Coloshield to protect the colo-anal anastomosis. The ring of the sterilised condom is sutured to the mucosal and submucosal layer of the proximal colon before completing the anastomosis. The condom is allowed to the exterior and transected with scissors. The device is expelled naturally from the anus between the 10th and 14th postoperative day.

4. Animal Models for Colonic Anastomosis

Although humans and animals may look different, at a physiological and anatomical level they are remarkably similar. Animals, from mice to monkeys, have the same organs and systems which perform the same functions in pretty much the same way. There are minor differences, but these are far outweighed by the similarities. The differences can give important clues about diseases and how they might be treated – for instance, if we knew why the mouse with muscular dystrophy suffers less muscle wasting than human patients, this might lead to a treatment for this debilitating and fatal disorder. It is settled that models never provide final answers of the original condition, but only offer approximation no single animal model can ever duplicate this original condition. Therefore, experimental science itself is the study of approximations and assimilation. To produce a good model, the best suited animal must be chosen regarding the physiologic and anatomic resemblance to man. Cost, availability, handling difficulty and housing requirements are important limitations which must all be considered when choosing the best models. A specific model is chosen because it is believed to be appropriate to the condition being investigated and is thought likely to respond in the same way as humans to the proposed treatment under investigation.

4.1. Animal Models in Biomedical Research

Models are widely used in all branches of physical, biological and social sciences. As defined in Oxford English Dictionary, a model in general is the representation of a real or actual object. In biomedical research, an animal model is defined as a living organism with an inherited, naturally acquired or induced pathological process trying to closely resemble the same phenomenon in man. Models are, thus, meant to mimic and it is not expected to be necessarily identical to the subject under investigation. In biomedical research, models allow the investigator to understand and investigate pathophysiological processes and the impact of intervention. The ultimate goal of experimental research using animal models is to solve problems in clinical practice and to develop new methods and approaches to the cure and alleviation of disease and disability.

4.2. Good Animal Model

Broadly speaking, not all animal species are useful for the purposes of biomedical research and the limitations of the models selected as well as the methodology involved must always be kept in mind. The optimal animal model should closely reproduce the disease in humans and therefore if possible the species with the closest anatomical and physiological resemblance to man should be used. On the other hand, a rare or exclusive animal should not be used, thus the model should be available to many researchers. The model should be economical and the anastomosis technically easy to perform. It should be reproducible with standardized interventions and measures. The animal should be easily handled by investigators and fit into an average institution.

4.3. Animals

4.3.1. The Mouse

The mouse has the advantages of being inexpensive, has a short life cycle, requires only limited space and is easily handled. As the rat, the mouse is not a strict herbivore, which means it has the ability to digest variable amounts of animal-derived food. With respect to the gastrointestinal tract, the mouse is comparable to man. Apart from lacking an appendix vermiformis, the mouse macroscopically has the same bowel segments as found in humans. Microscopically the intestinal wall consists of the same four layers as in humans: mucosa, submucosa, muscularis and serosa, with the epithelium of the colon consisting of columnar cells and many goblet cells. The mouse has been extensively used for research in oncology, toxicology, genetic engineering and to manufacture vaccines, antibodies and hormones, but few studies have used the mouse for surgical research. This might be due to the small size of the animal and thus small size of the organs, including the colon. The use of a microscope is necessary when performing a colonic anastomosis in the mouse. Mice and humans each have about 30,000 genes, yet only 300 are unique to either organism. Both even have genes for a tail, even though it's not "switched on" in humans. "About 99 percent of genes in humans have counterparts in the mouse," said Eric Lander, Director of the Whitehead Institute Center for Genomic Research in Cambridge, Massachusetts. "Eighty percent have identical, one-to-one counterparts."

4.3.2. The Rat

The rat is inexpensive, requires only limited space and is easy to handle. The rat has no gross anatomical peculiarities compared to man. The caecum is divided into an apex and a basal part by a slight constriction. When compared to the mouse, the larger size of the rat colon allows the anastomosis to be performed more easily and without the use of a microscope. Regarding the disadvantages, the rat is considered to be more resistant to infection compared to the mouse; however, this is a general consideration and has not been supported by studies on the issue. Moreover, one study found that young rats were protected against experimental fecal peritonitis by receiving maternal milk. Human beings do not have any specialized compartments in the digestive system because they, humans, are considered as omnivores, they eat both meat and vegetable or fruit plants. This means that all the support organs in their body have a special function to perform for our body. A rat digestive system has two major differences with that of a human. First, rats do not have a gallbladder. This is because they rarely take in large amount of fatty foods, thereby, making a gallbladder useless. Furthermore, rats have an enlarged large intestine, namely, the caecum. This helps them ferment the grains and seeds they take in, through the help of the bacteria inside thus, breaking down cellulose into nutrients.

4.3.3. The Rabbit

The rabbit requires only limited space, is easily handled and has a good size for surgical experiments, thus the relatively large size of the colon allows an anastomosis to be performed easily. For the disadvantage points of view, the rabbit is very susceptible to hypotension and dehydration during surgery, hence fluid therapy should be administered during the procedure. The rabbit has a very large caecum with a vermiform appendix and near the ileocolic valve there is an accumulation of lymphoid tissue which is called sacculus rotundus. This bears little resemblance with human anatomy. Rabbits are prone to abdominal adhesion formation and have been used as an experimental model for postsurgical adhesions in humans. Furthermore, the rabbit is more expensive than the mouse and rat.

4.3.4. The Dog

The variation in relative dimension of the large intestine is largely correlated with diet. The large intestine of carnivores is simple and very short, as its only purposes are to absorb salt and water. It is approximately the same diameter as the small intestine and, consequently, has a limited capacity to function as a reservoir. The colon is short and non-pouched. The muscle is distributed throughout the wall, giving the colon a smooth cylindrical appearance. Although a bacterial population is present in the colon of carnivores, its activities are essentially putrefactive.

In herbivores like horses and rabbits which depend largely on microbial fermentation, the large intestine is very large and complex. Omnivores like pigs and humans have a substantial large intestine, but nothing like that seen in herbivores.

Finally, carnivores such as dogs and cats have a simple and small large intestine. The dog is a pure carnivore. As all carnivores' digestive systems are the simplest. Despite overall anatomical differences, the colon and rectum of dogs are similar to those of man and the percentage of gastrointestinal tract to the whole body is similar in both dogs and humans and the caecum is relatively small and lacks an appendix vermiformis. The dog is easily handled but is expensive to purchase and maintain. In the past, they have frequently been used as surgical research models. However, growing public concern about using companion animals for research has forced scientists to use other species.

4.3.5. The Pig

Except for primates, the pig is the laboratory animal nearest to humans in terms of anatomy and physiology. This is also true for the gastrointestinal tract, which has very close resemblance to human physiology, digestive function and splanchnic blood flow characteristics. The length of the gastrointestinal tract is comparable to that of the adult human. Despite the spiral colon, a short transverse colon and a descending colon are accessible, but a true sigmoid flexure, as seen in humans, is not present in the pig. Thus, an intestinal anastomosis can be performed on the small intestine, transverse colon, descending colon, sigmoid colon and rectum.

Pigs are docile and trained easily and can be handled without difficulty. The relatively large size of the pig permits a variety of surgical interventions that are not possible in smaller animals and permits easy blood sampling, intravascular catheterization and endotracheal intubation. Pigs have been used extensively in human nutrition research. Their digestive system has some anatomical similarities and some differences compared to that of humans. Pigs and humans have comparable gastrointestinal tract (GIT) anatomy, morphology and physiology.

The GIT of a 30- to 40-kg pig is similar in total length to that of an adult human, and the relative sizes of the sections of human and pig GIT are alike with similar digestive physiology. Swine are true omnivores, as are humans. Furthermore, there is nearly complete agreement between humans and pigs in their dietary requirements for nutrients.

Regarding the main disadvantages, the pig is costly to purchase and maintain and requires more space for housing. The rapid growth rate of the pig makes it unsuitable for chronic experiments. Instead a mini-pig can be used if long-term follow-up is needed. Premedication and anesthesia in the pig is normally a more costly and complicated matter compared with rodents. The anatomy of the pig colon differs somewhat from man with a unique feature called the spiral colon. This structure consists of the cecum and the ascending colon coiled together into one structure. Mobilization and separation of the spiral colon is difficult, thus it is not amendable for anastomosis using standard techniques.

5. Telescoping Anastomosis

Researchers have repeatedly explored different methods in attempts to reduce operative time and improve functional results. In fact, Da Costa at 1931 stated that some 250 methods had been described for doing anastomoses. The basis of telescopic anastomosis is old, only the practical details of it have changed and improved. The telescoping or invaginating technique has been used but never widely acclaimed.

Throughout World Wide Web search for invaginating and telescoped anastomosis, the authors could find only few papers from 1957 to 2006 describing this technique. Gastrointestinal anastomoses by invagination were performed to restore gastroduodenal, ileocolic or colocolic continuity.

The telescopic anastomosis technique is successfully applied in clinical practice for reconstruction of gastrectomy and esophageal resection. Huan-wei Chen and his colleagues at 2008 used the pancreaticojejunal anastomosis by invagination to a depth of 4 cm into the jejunum, and the invagination is secured by two sutures at the superior and inferior parts of the pancreatic stump. They reported that healing of the pancreaticojejunal invagination can be facilitated by jejunal mucosal cauterization, which prevents the secretions from the jejunal mucosa from becoming trapped in the jejunum–pancreatic interface, and which also induces inflammation to promote healing after invagination.

By invagination, pancreatic juice from the main pancreatic duct and pancreatic stump drain into the jejunum. The results of pancreaticojejunostomy invaginating anastomotic technique showed a zero leakage/fistula rate, a low incidence of morbidity, and a low mortality rate. The vascular anastomoses by invagination were also reported in clinical and experimental studies.

The adventitia of the proximal part of the anastomosed artery is usually and subsequently prepared and removed. The anastomosis is completed where one end is invaginated into the other and is fixed firmly. Rickard and others at 2011 performed their experimental vascular anastomosis by invaginating the smaller vessel inside the larger in the management of size discrepancy and they found the invaginating anastomosis being faster to perform and produces comparable patency in a rat model.

5.1. Technique

5.1.1. Anesthesia

The animal should be premedicated preoperatively by intramuscular administration of chlorpromazine hydrochloride 1 mg/kg body weight 20-30 minutes prior to surgery. Induction of anesthesia is achieved by intravenous administration of sodium thiopental 2.5 % solution 20-30 mg/kg via a 20 gauge intravenous cannula. Anesthesia is maintained during the operation by further small doses of thiopental sodium.

5.1.2. Surgical Procedure

The skin of the abdomen is shaved, and antisepsis is performed using povidone-iodine and a midline skin incision of approximately 10 cm length is made below the umbilicus to the symphysis pubis. After reaching the abdominal cavity, the left colon is exposed. Division of the sigmoid colon is done between two non-crushing intestinal clamps and the bowel continuity is restored using invaginating anastomosis technique as illustrated in the diagrammatic representation [figure1].

Four invaginating stay sutures are performed. The first stitch should start10 mm from the edge of the distal segment at the position of 12 o'clock (serosa-mucosa), and then passes through the mucosa-serosa, just to the cut edge of the proximal segment. Thereafter, the needle is reintroduced again into serosa-mucosa and emerged just to the cut edge (the same distance) of the proximal segment.

The needle, thereafter, passes to the mucosa-serosa of the distal segment, 10 mm apart from and parallel to the first bite. The other three stay sutures are performed in the same manner at the position of 6, 3 and 9 o'clock from the colonic circumference.

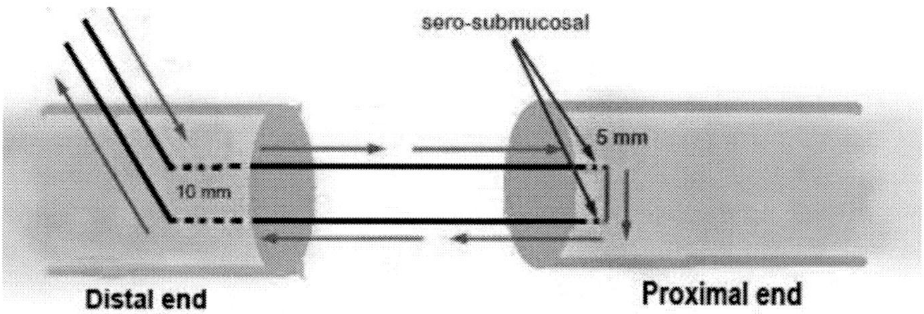

Figure 1. A diagrammatic illustration showing how the proximal segment is invaginated into the distal.

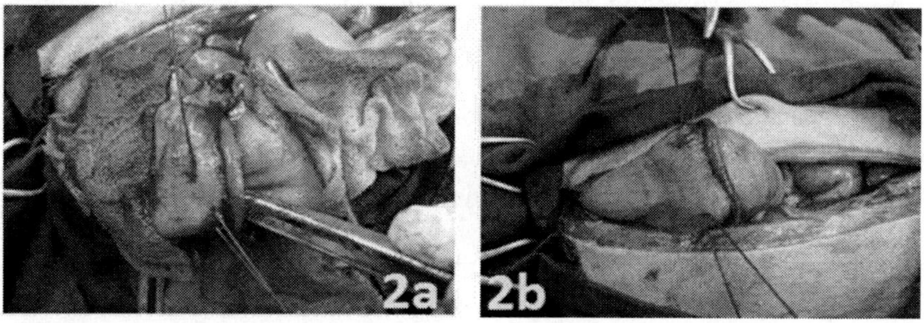

Figure 2 a. b. The start of invaginating the proximal segment into the distal one. The rim of the distal segment is just being sutured to the serosa of the proximal one aiming to complete the invagination.

By tying these sutures, invagination of the proximal segment into the distal one is invited. Between these four sutures, the rim of the distal segment is sutured to the serosa of the proximal one [figure 2 a, b]. At first, invagination length of the proximal segment was 40-50 mm as reported by Linn and his colleagues at 1968 then being as short as 10 mm in the present author's technique and in an experimental work of same interest done by Szucs and his colleagues at 2003. The previous experimental procedures of invagination were done either without mucosal dissection or with dissection of distal bowel mucosa using single layer of interrupted sutures but in the present technique, the author used four invaginating sutures to securely fix the proximal end to into the distal, a maneuver that is lacking in those previous works.

5.1. Outcome

The technical feasibility and efficacy of the telescoping intestinal anastomosis are confirmed through the stability of the induced anastomosis. Both the external and internal features at the site of anastomotic lines as well as the microscopic configuration of the invaginating colocolic anastomosis and its efficacy in creating strong bowel continuity, all are at the level of high satisfaction as reported by many researchers.

5.2.1. Patency of the Anastomosis

a. Anastomotic leak:

Colorectal anastomotic leakage remains one of the most feared post-operative complications and long-term functional outcome might be adversely affected by anastomotic leakage. The safety of an intestinal anastomosis is usually measured by its complication rate, especially the incidence of anastomotic leakage.

Some leaks presents in a dramatic fashion early in the postoperative period, leaving little doubt about the diagnosis. However, many other leaks present relatively late in the postoperative period in a far more subtle fashion, and can be difficult to distinguish from other postoperative infectious complications.

Clinical and occult radiological anastomotic leakage may reach up to 40 %, depending on the height of anastomosis, the type of operation, and the experience of the surgeon.

As regard the clinical picture, patients classically develop agonizing abdominal pain, tachycardia, high fevers, and abdominal rigidity with or without hemodynamic instability.

In these cases, urgent exploration for peritoneal washout and fecal diversion is required. Furthermore, anastomotic leakage has been associated with increased local recurrence and diminished survival after colorectal cancer surgery. Radiologic imaging is usually required; even then, the diagnosis may be elusive or at least uncertain. Imaging study using the soluble material; gastrografin would detect any evidence of leak or perianastomotic abscess formation or perianastomotic collection closely related to the anastomotic line [figure 3 a, b, and c].

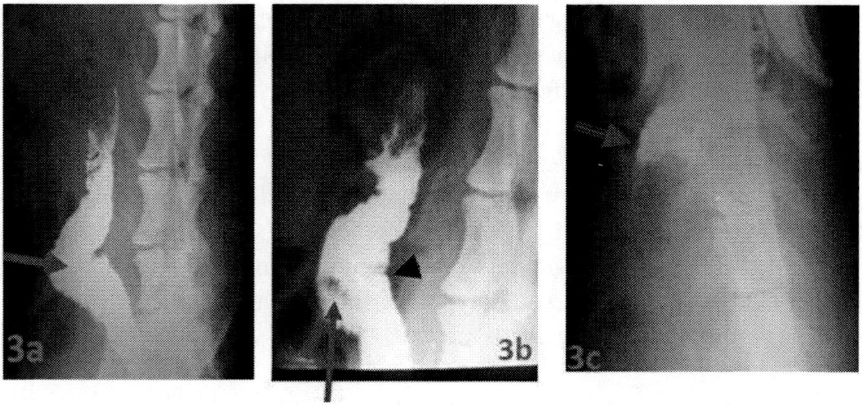

Figure 3.a, b and c. Imaging study using the soluble material; gastrografin revealed no evidence of leak or perianastomotic abscess [3a: telescoping] and evidence of a perianastomotic collection closely related to the anastomotic line. The post-evacuation film showed free residence of the contrast in the peritoneal cavity [3b, c: end to end].

b. External appearance of the anastomosis:

The author in his previous experimental studies advocated a descriptive scaling system for evaluating the external anastomotic configuration. On gross examination, anastomotic lines are rated as good if there is no evidence of leak or stenosis. Fair rating is assigned if there is stenosis only but not leak and a rating of poor is reserved for any evidence of leak with or without stenosis. Stenosis or stricture is considered where the proximal segment of the anastomosis is twice larger than that of the distal segment. Benign anastomotic strictures frequently complicate colonic resections and occur in 3-30% of post colorectal anastomosis according to varied definitions. This anastomotic stricture is considered to be related to factors such as ischemia or leakage and suture technique. The author in his previous reports noticed that invaginating and telescoped anastomosis is usually associated with low incidence of anastomotic stenosis when compared with end to end single layer anastomosis regarding the good and fair rating of external examination of anastomoses.

c. Internal appearance of the anastomosis:

The interior aspect of the anastomotic areas in the telescoping technique is checked for mucosal ulcer, perianastomotic ischaemia or necrosis and the fate of the invaginated segment. According to the author's experience, the naked eye examination of the interior aspect of the anastomotic areas revealed that there is no mucosal ulcer in animals of telescoping anastomosis and good mucosal creeping around the anastomotic lines. Regarding the perianastomotic ischaemia or necrosis, the anastomotic field is completely without ischaemia or necrosis and the invaginated segments are completely disappeared under cover of the mucosal creeping.

5.2.2. Manometric Evaluation

A simple manometer is usually used to evaluate the anastomotic integrity. This simple manometer is in the form of a graduated scale connected to an air insufflator. Bursting pressure is the minimal force exerted to cause anastomotic perforation. Bursting pressure is used as a quantitative measure to grade the strength of colonic anastomosis.

a. Intraoperative manometric evaluation

Through a small colotomy opening, the tube of the manometer is introduced into the lumen and fitted to the wall by purse string suture using 2/0 silk. The proximal and distal colonic ends are occluded by noncrushing intestinal clamps while the anastomotic lines should be in between. Measuring the intraoperative manometric evaluation in previous experiments done by the author denoted that the invaginating technique is more potent when compared with other techniques such as the interrupted single-layer serosubmucosal anastomosis and showed that this power is due to the anastomotic technique itself not for collagen formation or the invaginated part and this observed point came in agreement with other studies of same interest.

b. Postoperative manometric evaluation

The postoperative bursting pressure is usually measured by dissecting the colonic segment carrying the anastomotic site en block and one end of the resected segment is tied off while the other is tied over the tube connected to the pressure transducer of the manometer. The resected segment together with the connecting tube should then be emerged in a clean water bath to detect any air leakage when burst occurred. By means of the manometer, the intraluminal pressure should increase by 10 mmHg over 10 second at intervals of 10 seconds also. This pressure has been found to increase rapidly in the early postoperative period, reaching 60% of the strength of the surrounding bowel by three to four days and 100% by one week. However, it is stated that after establishing the healing process within 14 – 21 days of the experiments, the manometric values are increased more than that in the early postoperative values and there is no statistically significant difference among the bursting pressures of the various anastomoses performed. In 1887, Halsted discovered that the submucosa provides the majority of the tensile strength and the bulk of collagen is contained within this layer. During the first postoperative days, anastomotic strength is limited, and hence the risk of wound failure is greatest, as collagen breakdown increases. Early anastomotic strength is therefore dependent on any anastomotic technique reserving the holding capacity of existing collagen, until a large amount of new collagen can be synthesized by both fibroblasts and smooth muscle cells. Postoperatively, anastomosis will be weak for one or two days until this occurs. The mean values of bursting pressure of the anastomoses in animals with the invaginating technique are significantly higher than those of other techniques in the freshly constructed anastomoses and before any attempt at healing activity when the bursting pressure was checked intraoperatively or in vitro. When the anastomotic stability is studied after three weeks, the postoperative manometric study of the bursting pressure values in the invaginating and other techniques usually shows no statistical significant difference despite still higher in case of the invaginating technique and this fact is attributed to establishing the healing process within two three weeks of the experiments and new collagen deposition.

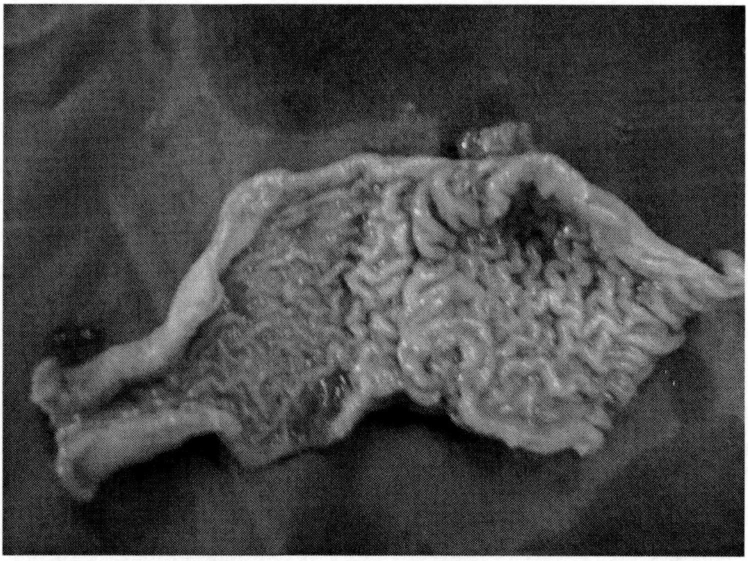

Figure 4. A postoperative photograph showed the interior aspect of the anastomotic areas with no mucosal ulcers and with good mucosal creeping. The invaginated segment was completely disappeared under cover of the mucosal creeping.

5.2.3. Detection of Adhesion Formation

Adhesions are a common, and an inevitable consequence of serosal repair and the process of adhesion formation involve the absence or modification of fibrinolytic mechanisms and migration and proliferation of a variety of cell types, including inflammatory cells, mesothelial cells, and fibroblasts and the degree of its severity is proportional to the magnitude of surgical trauma. Adhesion formation is part of the innate peritoneal defense mechanism in peritonitis. Adhesion formation is usually divided according to severity as previously described by the author in his experimental works on rats and dogs into localized, moderate and extensive. Localized adhesion represents a single band of adhesion or in the form of perianastomotic adhesion formed of small intestinal loops or omentum while the moderate adhesion represents the form of perianastomotic adhesion formed of small intestinal loops or omentum plus a single band extending between the abdominal surface of the wound and the omentum or adherence of two loops of gut. The extensive adhesion was detected between the small intestine, omentum and the anastomotic site. Anastomotic leak and abscess formation are well-known complications after surgery associated with fibrinous adhesions As the leakage in invaginating anastomoses is nearly completely absent in the telescoping anastomosis, it is logic to be associated with less total adhesion score than any other technique.

5.2.4. Histopathological Study

According to others studies, there was considerably more suture-line inflammation, edema, micro-abscess formation, mucosal ulceration and pericolic inflammation of the fat in the one-layer, two-layer, and stapled anastomoses than in the telescoping anastomosis. In concordance with these finding, the invaginating and telescoping anastomosis according to the author's previous reports, usually states that good regenerative activity of mucosal healing and good effacing between the two cut edges of the mucosal epithelium are more evident. Logically, when the mucosal layer is included in surgical sutures, certain degree of ischemic necrosis always develops, that delays the intestinal healing, prolongs inflammation and produces excessive cellular proliferation and this surgical and histopsthological fact is actually observed in the one-layer, two-layer, and stapled anastomoses with excessive inflammation more than the invaginating and telescoping anastomosis where inflammatory cell exudate usually shows only focal aggregation of lymphocytes. Fibroblast activity occurs mainly during the third phase of the healing process. Fibroblasts migrate to the anastomotic site from surrounding tissues and start the collagen production. As a good parameter of healing in the invaginating and telescoping anastomosis according to the author's previous experimental works, the fibroblastic activity showed good regenerative power filling the gap between the two cut ends of muscularis mucosa more than the conventional single-layer end to end anastomosis. Neoangiogenesis is an important element of the healing process and the healing power is directly proportional to the heaviness of neoangiogenesis. Despite statistically insignificant, the whole histopathological score including neo-capillary formation with good vascularity was observed in the two group of the present study.

6. Further Reading

Historical Background

Coolman BR. Ehrhart N, Marretta SM. Historical perspective of intestinal anastomosis in veterinary surgery. *Compend. Contin. Educ. Pract. Vet.* 2000: 22:232.

Nasirkhan MU, Abir F, Longo W, Kozol R. Anastomotic disruption after large bowel resection. *World J. Gastroenterol.* 2006 April 28;12(16): 2497-2504.

Nuhu A, Jah A. Acute Sigmoid Volvulus in a West African Population. *Ann. Afr. Med.* 2010;9(2):86-90.

Saber A. Ancient Egyptian Surgical Heritage. *Journal of Investigative Surgery,* 2010, 23, (6): 327-334.

Techniques of Colonic Anastomosis

Mortensen NFand Ashraf S. ACS Surgery: Principles And Practice 5 Gastrointestinal Tract And Abdomen 29 Intestinal Anastomosis. DC Becker Inc, 2008.

Hsiao W C, Young K C, Wang S T, Lin P W. Incisional hernia after laparotomy: randomised comparison between early-absorbable and late-absorbable suture materials. *World J. Surg.* 2000; 24: 747-751.

Puleo S, Sofia M, Trovato MA, Pesce A, Portale TR, Russello D, La Greca G. Ileocolonic anastomosis: preferred techniques in 999 patients. multicentric study. *Surg. Today.* 2012 Oct 31. [Epub ahead of print].

Ho YH, Ashour MA. Techniques for colorectal anastomosis. *World J. Gastroenterol.* 2010 : 7; 16(13): 1610–1621.

Dahl DM, and McDougal WS. Use of Intestinal Segments in Urinary Diversion. In: Wein: Campbell-Walsh Urology, 10th. Ed. Saunders, 2011:2411-2449.

Anastomotic Line Protection

Pommergaard HC, Achiam MP, Rosenberg J. External coating of colonic anastomoses: a systematic review. *Int. J. Colorectal. Dis.* 2012 Oct;27(10):1247-58.

Hoeppner J, Crnogorac V, Marjanovic G, Jüttner E, Keck T, Weiser HF, Hopt UT. Small intestinal submucosa for reinforcement of colonic anastomosis. *Int. J. Colorectal. Dis.* 2009 ;24(5):543-50.

Morks AN, Havenga K, Ploeg RJ. Can intraluminal devices prevent or reduce colorectal anastomotic leakage: A review. *World J. Gastroenterol.* 2011 :28; 17(40): 4461–4469.

Bolzam-Nascimento R, Coy CS, Pereira YE, Leal RF, Reis RC, Mantovani M, Ayrizono Mde L, Chung WF, Fagundes JJ. Influence of omentoplasty on colonic anastomosis in animals submitted to hemorrhagic shock in rats. *Acta Cir. Bras*. 2009 May-Jun;24(3):233-8.

Pommergaard HC, Rosenberg J, Schumacher-Petersen C, Achiam MP. Choosing the Best Animal Species to Mimic Clinical Colon Anastomotic Leakage in Humans: A Qualitative Systematic Review. *Eur. Surg. Res.* 2011;47:173-181 (DOI: 10.1159/000330748).

Animal Models for Colonic Anastomosis

Gandarillas M and Bas F. The domestic pig (Sus scrofa domestica) as a model for evaluating nutritional and metabolic consequences of bariatric surgery practiced on morbid obese humans Cien. *Inv. Agr*. 2009;36(2): 163-176.

Pommergaard HC, Rosenberg J, Schumacher-Petersen C, Achiam MP. Choosing the Best Animal Species to Mimic Clinical Colon Anastomotic Leakage in Humans: A Qualitative Systematic Review. *Eur. Surg. Res*. 2011;47:173-181 (DOI: 10.1159/000330748).

Saber A: Effect of Intergel versus Honey in Intraperitoneal Adhesion Prevention and Colonic Anastomotic Healing: A Comparative

Experimental Study in Rats. Thesis (M.D). Suez-Canal University: Faculty of Medicine; 2005.

Telescoping Anastomosis

Burson LC, Berliner SD, Strauss RJ, Katz P, Wise L. Telescoping anastomosis of the colon: a comparative study. *Dis. Colon. Rectum*. 1979 ;22(2):111-6.

Linn BS, Reisman TM, Yurt RW, Polk HC Jr. Intestinal anastomosis by invagination: a historical review of a "new" technic with controlled study of its potential. *Ann. Surg*. 1968 ;167(3):393-8.

Rickard RF, Engelbrecht GH, Hudson DA. Experimental investigation of two techniques of arterial microanastomosis used to manage a small-to-large diameter discrepancy. *J. Plast. Reconstr. Aesthet. Surg*. 2011;64(8):1088-95.

Saber A, Shekidef MH, Fatih H A. Telescoping Colonic Anastomosis in Dogs: Gross and Microscopic Configurations. *Arch. Clin. Exp. Surg.* doi: 10.5455/aces.20120218120802.

Saber A, Shekidef MH, Fatih H A. Invaginating versus single layer colonic anastomosis: A comparative study in dogs. W*orld Journal of Colorectal Surgery* [Accepted].

Saber A. Invaginating versus single layer colonic anastomosis: A comparative study in dogs ".21st World Congress of the International Association of Surgeons, *Gastroenterologists and Oncologists* (IASGO), November, 2011, Tokyo. Japan.

Szucs G, Tóth I, Barna T, Bráth E, Gyáni K, Mikó I Operation technique and healing process of telescopic ileocolostomy in dogs. *Acta Vet. Hung.* 2003;51(4):539-50.

In: Anastomoses ISBN: 978-1-62618-657-6
Editors: F. King, McKineley A. Malloy © 2013 Nova Science Publishers, Inc.

Chapter IV

Expandable Devices for Easier, Quicker and More Efficient Aortic-Prosthesis Anastomosis[1]

Stefano Nazari
Foundation Alexis Carrel, Italy

Abstract

Open thoracic aorta prosthetic substitution still carries significant mortality and serious complications risk, in particular to CNS. Risk is mostly correlated to the length of clamping/circulatory arrest time, i.e. essentially to the time required for vascular anastomosis construction.

We developed devices for easier, quicker and more efficient aortic-prosthesis anastomosis based on a new working principle: i.e. compression of vascular stump between inner (nitinol wireframe) and outer structures (external ligature or nitinol wireframe) instead of sewing with full-thickness perforation of the vessel wall.

The device consists of loops of nitinol wires, wrapped within a Dacron fabric and connected to a prosthesis end (Type I and III). The nitinol wire loops can be expanded and tightened by activating a removable guide in such a way that device varies its diameter, while maintaining a regular cylindrical shape. This allows the easy and quick insertion of the retracted device into the vascular stump and then its

[1] EACTS-Tecno College Award Nominee 2012, Barcellona Oct 27-31, 2012.

expansion to perfectly fit with the vessel diameter. Haemostasis and permanent device fixation are provided by external ligature/suture.

Three main models (Type I, II and III) applying the same working mechanism, but with different configurations, allow to fit with all aorta segments as well as special conditions of use.

Device type I, previously connected with a tube graft end, is used for the first anastomosis, either proximal or distal; device type II is then used for the second anastomosis after having tailored the graft tube at its appropriate length.

Device type III is ideally used for anastomosis in dissection cases, allowing in particular to include even the concavity of arch. Single graft layer type I devices for small diameters (6-14 mm) can be used for supraortic trunks.

The regularly expandable configuration of the ring device allows to solve all the insertion, positioning and stability problems of the 70ies intraluminal prosthesis. That makes performing anastomosis a very simple task, which can be carried out in seconds vs the 10-15 min per anastomosis at best required with hand suture.

The aortic wall being not perforated by the suture, the coupling is immediately blood-thigh ("air-tight" in fact!) and then independent by the integrity of the physiological coagulation mechanisms.

In summary favorable effects on complications rate, particularly in aortic arch substitution, related to circulatory arrest, hypothermia and CNS perfusion and dissection layers reconstructions can be expected due to:

1. 1-dramatic reduction of the time required for completing aortic prosthetic anastomosis because of a) great simplification of anastomosis technique, which is performed at once with b) double strip graft vascular stump buttressing and c)"air-tight" sealing dissection layers re-approximation
2. 2-easy and quick supraortic trunks anastomosis previously prepared on the main tube graft.

Anastomosis immediate blood-tightness not dependent on coagulation integrity may predictably decrease intra- and postoperative blood losses. Use of these devices may also enhance mininvasive access in prosthetic open substitution of any aortic segments.

1. Introduction

1.1. Background

1.1.1. The Beginnings

Vascular surgery was quite obviously conditioned by the development and evolution of the techniques for vascular anastomosis, started around the beginning of the past century. Apart in fact from few episodic and lucky clinical cases of lateral laceration repair as well as many experimental endeavors of vascular suture, accurately described and illustrated in a detailed historical Italian review [49], before that point in time vascular surgery clinical practice was substantially confined to vascular ligature.

In 1900 Erwin Payr reported to the German Surgical Society results on animal experiments of the apparently first device for vascular anastomosis, which is essentially based on external ligature of vascular stumps over a rigid and absorbable magnesium ring [35], thus trying to adapting to surgery a method already universally used for coupling floppy/elastic tubing (Figure 1).

In spite of its elegance (intima-to-intima facing, absorbable magnesium ring) one of its implicit mechanical limits was already outlined in the original report: elastic retraction of the vascular wall when clamped significantly reduces its diameter, thus making quite difficult to put in place a rigid ring of appropriate diameter.

In those very years Alexis Carrel, as well as many others in fact [47], was focusing his attention on suture techniques, already currently adopted in the gastrointestinal tract, and was able to realize blood-tight, low thrombogenic vascular anastomoses by careful refinements of the needles, threads and techniques for their use [7, 8], thus establishing the standard technique of vascular surgery.

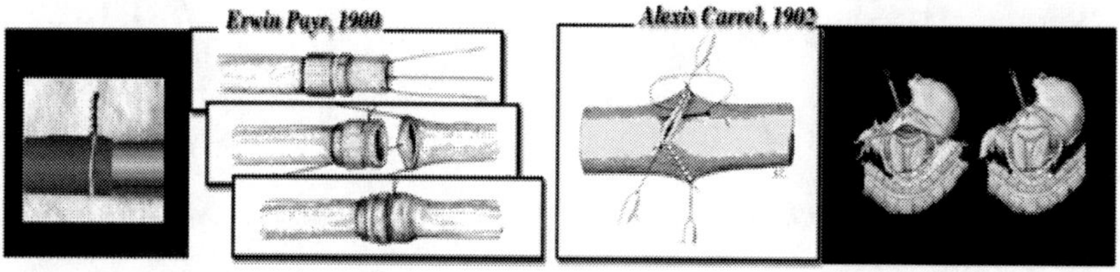

Figure 1. Payr and Carrel pioneering techniques. Payr first reported device for vascular anastomosis substantially derived from elaboration of the common method for rubber tubing connection (left square) while Carrel triangulation was apparently derived from refinements of gastrointestinal suture (right square).

Although technically demanding, its versatility allowed to deal with virtually all clinical occurrences, from large aortic to microsurgical anastomosis, so that the many and significant improvements in needles (i.e. curved, atraumatic), threads (i.e. polypropylene) and surgical technique (i.e. parachute, etc.) developed throughout more than a century could not break the ideal line linking the Nobel prize acknowledged (1912) Carrel original work with today clinical practice.

Interestingly enough for more than a century vascular anastomosis technique research moved forward, very slowly to say the truth, with occasional brief clinical applications essentially along these two basic principles only, with the possible exception of gluing based methods.

1.2. Vascular Staplers

It was in fact substantially a technological evolution of the Carrel coupling principle (full thickness wall stump stitching) that gave origin, around the middle of the past century, to stapling devices with the aim of automating the anastomoses.

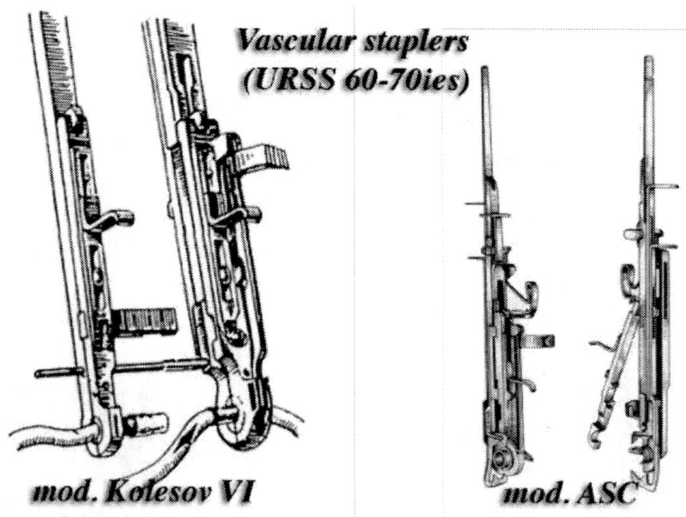

Figure 2. Models of URSS vascular staplers (1960-70). Similar bulky and cumbersome devices were also realized at that time in Canada, USA and Japan.

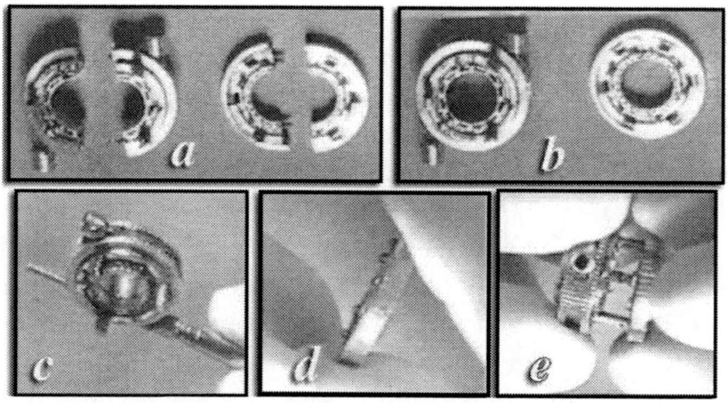

Figure 3. Vascular stapler for reducing warm ischemia in organ transplantation. With our model each stapler end can be mounted on donor and recipient by independent surgical teams without care for reciprocal orientation, being the maximal possible vascular axis torsion ≤30°. Activating guide-wire is connected just immediately before firing (24). Video at http://www.fondazionecarrel.org/nazarichaptervideo.html.

However, while stapling devices have long since allowed standardization and simplification of digestive tract circular anastomosis, despite extensive research (see exhaustive reviews: Tesauro 1967 [42]; Tesauro and Persico 1979 [43]), including our own [24], the stapling principle has so far failed to be of significant use for vascular anastomosis, which remains substantially the only basic surgical task still to be automated.

The 60-70ies stapling devices (Figure 2) have all quite cumbersome and heavy configurations in particular in relation to the delicate structure of the quite small diameter vessel to which they were intended to be used in those years.

With this in mind first of all we tried to simplify the procedure by severing the stapling device (Figure 3) from the activating handle, which in our device consisted in a flexible, camera-type, firing guide-wire that could be connected to the stapler after its coupling with vascular stumps just before firing (Figure 4, c), at the more convenient of the two opposite sides connecting spots (Figure 3). Moreover the two stapler parts were designed in such a way that each one could be mounted on the vascular stump by independent surgical teams without taking care for their reciprocal orientation; the connectors of the two parts of the stapler in fact allowed to limit the maximal possible vascular axis torsion to 30°.

One of the crucial points mechanically implicit in any vascular stapler model is related to the requirement of temporary fixation of the vascular stumps to the device ends in preparation for the anastomosis.

The vascular stump link to each device end in fact must be, on one side, strong enough to be maintained during device manipulation for ends coupling but, on the other side, should be weak enough to be easily released after stapler firing, to allow the device ends to be divided and removed.

Being our stapler ideated for use in organ transplantation to reduce the warm ischemic phase, we could solve this problem by temporarily suturing vascular stumps to the stapler end by single thread on predisposed little rings (Figure 3, d); this can be done independently by the donor surgical team at back table to one stapler end (Figure 4, a) and by the recipient team to the other stapler end, without interfering with time of critical surgical phases. When the donor organ is at the recipient operative table (Figure 4, b) the two stapler ends can be easily and quickly connected and the stapler fired (Figure 4, c). Only when the circulation is resumed the sutures temporarily connecting the vascular stumps to the stapler ends can be sectioned and the device removed (Figure 4, d) without impacting on the organ warm ischemia time.

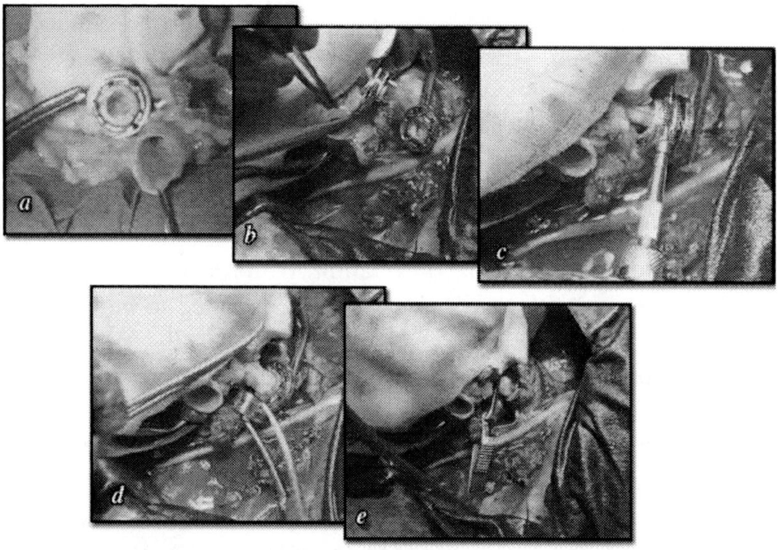

Figure 4. Vascular stapler for reducing warm ischemia in experimental lung transplantation. In a canine model of left single lung transplantation one stapler end was applied on donor pulmonary artery at back table (a) and the other by the recipient surgical team; then the two ends are quickly connected together (b), the firing wire connected and activated (c). After having sectioned the two sutures linking the vascular stumps to the device ends, the two stapler parts were divided and removed (d) and anastomosis checked (e) still preventing graft perfusion until atrial connection was established [24]. Video at http://www.fondazionecarrel.org/nazarichaptervideo.html.

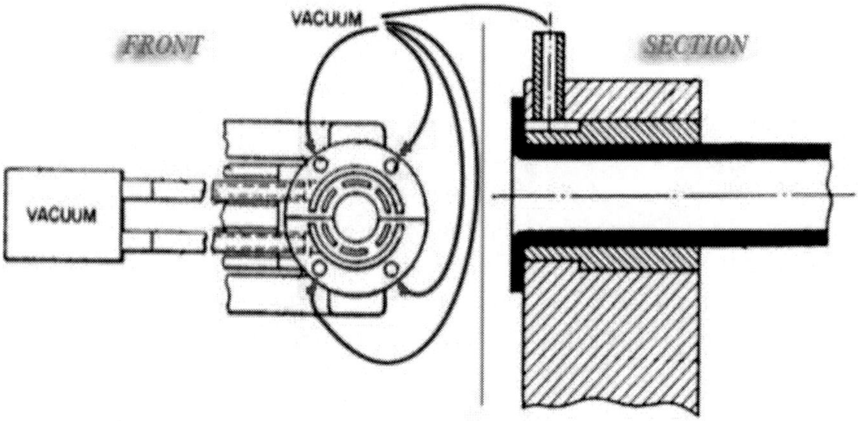

Figure 5. Kolesov VI vacuum assisted vascular stapler. To temporarily connect coronary artery stumps to the stapler ends, vacuum is applied to the predisposed device whose surface then sucks and holds the vascular wall (red arrows).

An elegant technical solution to this problem was provided by V. Kolesov [18, 19], credited for the first LIMA-coronary artery by pass [20] and the first surgeon to have clinically used coronary stapling device. He devised to realize this vascular stump-stapler end temporary link by applying vacuum to each device end whose surface was appropriately predisposed (Figure 5, red arrows) thus sucking and holding the vascular stump in position. This seems a simple and effective method that can ideally fit with the surgical need and possibly solve this part of the vascular stapler problems.

In synthesis however, even though research restlessly continue to produce new prototypes, the apparently unavoidable critical point is that the intrinsic manual surgical skill required to put in position and operate any stapler on the delicate vascular structure didn't yet (can't?) result in a easier, simpler, quicker and more efficient task than standard hand suture, even when its use is for very large diameter vessel only [39].

1.3. Intraluminal Ringed Prosthesis

In the 1970–1980s, a simplified Payr concept was revived with the introduction of intraluminal ringed prostheses, whose use in aortic substitution was quite extensively reported (Figure 6) [21, 3, 11].

The reasons for their clinical failure have been numerous. Mechanical facts implicit in the method (Figure 7) are related both to the elastic retraction of the vessel when is clamped, already outlined in the Payr report [35], and to the floppy consistency of the vascular wall that requires a further significant gap to be left between the clamped internal aortic wall and the external ring diameter to allow the ring to be easily slipped into the vascular stump without friction.

Accordingly a ringed prosthesis with a diameter significantly smaller than appropriate must be used to keep the cross-clamping time shorter than that attainable with manual suturing [26].

Thus when the aorta is re-perfused, the resulting discrepancy between perfused vascular stump and intraluminal ring diameter generates conditions greatly favoring coupling instability (Figure 7, C); moreover it can be argued that possible generation of systolic movements of the aortic wall at ligature hinge may potentially cause mechanical friction/erosion and thus eventually rupture. (Figure 7, D).

Many other inappropriate constructive features of those devices were probably responsible for their eventual failure. Thus the rigid ring was too short to be easily identified from outside the aorta, making very difficult the appropriate positioning of the external ligature; moreover the groove shape and dimension were inappropriate to maintain coupling stability.

This latter point offers the occasion for some important consideration. Vascular anastomosis must guarantee two essential mechanical facts: haemostatic sealing and stability of the coupling. This may seem a self-evident, unnecessary distinction since both are obviously provided at once by the standard hand suture; not so however with the “Payr” coupling principle, which is at basis of 70-80ies intraluminal prosthesis as well as of our expandable device.

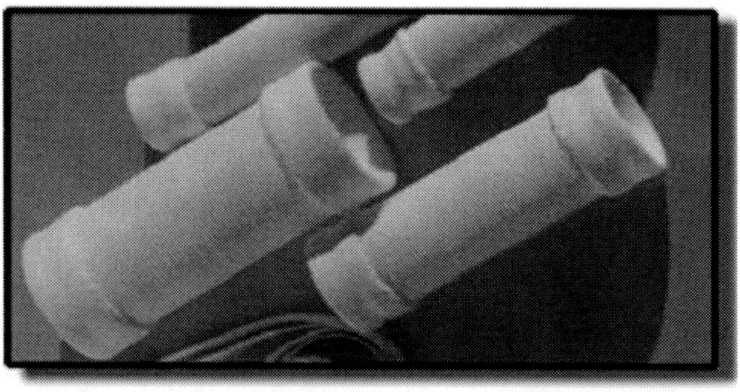

Figure 6. Intraluminal ringed prosthesis. Aortic anastomotic device commercially available (FDA) in 70-90ies.

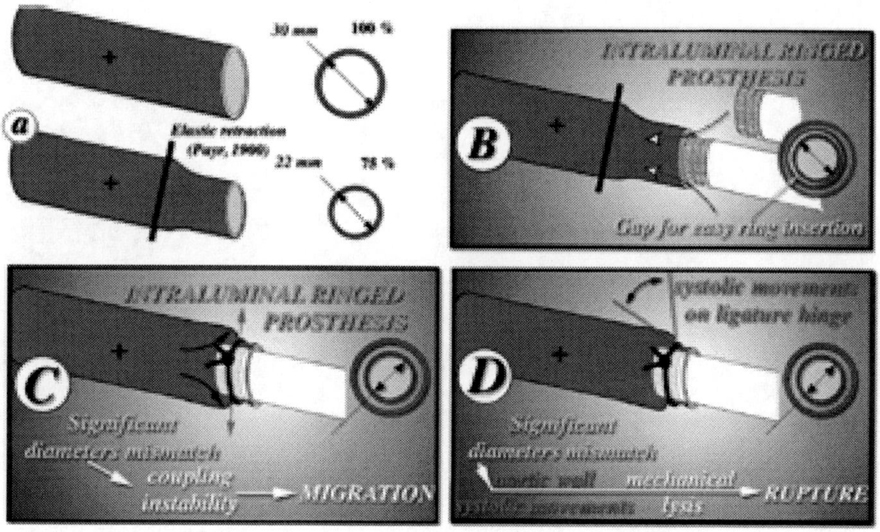

Figure 7. Facts related to intraluminal ringed prosthesis (Payr type coupling). When the vessel is clamped there is a significant reduction of the stump diameter due to its elastic retraction (a); moreover because of the floppy consistency of the vascular wall a significant gap (b) must be left between outer ring and inner stump diameter for a rapid positioning. When blood flow is resumed the resulting significant diameter mismatch (c) generates conditions for coupling instability and device dislocation. It may also be hypothesized that systolic movements on ligature hinge (d) may generate mechanical erosion and possibly rupture.

While in fact to achieve haemostatic seal is sufficient to apply on the vascular stump external surface a pressure equal or just exceeding the blood pressure, that pressure or even a much higher pressure may not be enough to prevent the vascular stump from slipping off from the inner sleeve (Figure 8, large square).

Then means to increase friction (i.e. groove or hooks, etc.) between the opposing surfaces or to permanently link them together (i.e. full thickness stitches) must be put in place to prevent vascular stump from sliding off. Although this was soon recognized (and solved!) by gardeners since many years (Figure 8, upper right square), the failure of the 70-80ies intraluminal prosthesis may have been caused also by underestimation (Figure 8, lower right square) of this not irrelevant detail.

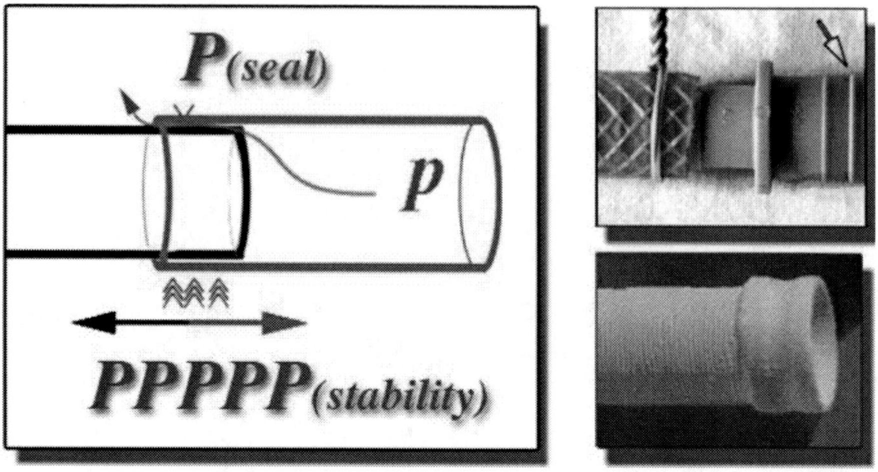

Figure 8. Haemostasis and stability in Payr coupling type. While hemostasis can be achieved by applying an external pressure ≥ blood pressure, even much higher pressure may not prevent the stump from slipping over the inner sleeve and split apart (larger square). Grooves on the inner sleeve outer surface can prevent dislocation only if appropriately dimensioned and shaped (right upper square). Intraluminal prosthesis groove appears inappropriate in deepness, length and shape to keep coupling stability (right lower square).

1.4. Endovascular Surgery

In the last decade of the past century, preceded by various pioneering works [9, 45, 46] and popularized by J.C Parodi clinical reports [33, 34], endovascular techniques burst into clinical vascular surgery, allowing prosthesis positioning into the aneurysm and excluding it from blood stream without open surgery. This provided a less invasive and lower complications rate therapeutic tool that allowed cure for patients previously not amenable to open surgery for age, general conditions or associated risk factors. First successfully popularized in infrarenal aortic aneurysm, techniques and materials continuing improvements allowed endovascular prosthetic substitution of virtually all segments of aorta, including arch, even though sometime with hybrid procedures [6, 2, 41, 13].

It is not the aim of this chapter to describe, even summarily, the historical evolution of these techniques, but rather to try to outline the proved facts of these new therapeutic tools at this point in time. While obviously technological evolution will further extend indications and improvements in clinical results, superiority of endovascular method vs open surgery at this point in time was conclusively proved in infrarenal aortic aneurysms and in uncomplicated, non genetic, isolated descending aorta aneurysms [15]. An interesting result of several recent studies [44, 12, 38] showed that, despite a two-thirds decrease in 30-day operative mortality rate after endovascular abdominal aortic aneurism repair (EVAR) compared with open repair, the all-cause mortality curves converge during the first 2-3 years thereafter, with no significant difference in all-cause mortality beyond this time. A recent study [4] seems to indicate that more cardiovascular deaths in the EVAR patients group contribute to the convergence in all-cause mortality during the first 2 years.

Quite wide clinical experience however already showed that endovascular procedures cannot protect from spinal chord ischemia and consequent paraplegia in extended descending aorta prosthetic substitution. It has been hypothesized that this could be due, at least in some case, to the fact that while endoprosthesis immediately prevents intercostal branches to be physiologically perfused, cannot prevent, at least for a certain time in the initial phase, backwards blood flow into the space between endoprosthesis and aortic wall, thus generating conditions for a blood flow "steal" from perfusion of the spinal chord [17].

Last but not least overall recent USA Nationwide Inpatient Sample data 2006-2007 review [15] showed that only 23% (2,563/11,669) of ideal candidate to endovascular treatment (uncomplicated, elective descending aortic aneurysms) underwent endovascular procedure (TEVAR), while the remaining 77% (9,106/11,669) still underwent open surgical repair.

These facts prompted us to consider new strategies against aortic aneurysm based on new tools we developed for its treatment.

2. New Expandable Devices for Easier, Quicker and More Efficient Open Surgery for Large Thoracic or Thoracoabdominal Aneurysms

Even though endovascular techniques will continuously gain wider indications for prosthetic substitution of the aorta, more complex cases will always remain in which open surgery is the only or the best option. Moreover while acute aortic syndrome is obviously spread throughout the territory, only highly specialized centers can offer endovascular techniques as an emergency measure; current data show that vast majority (77%) of uncomplicated, non genetic elective descending aorta aneurisms still underwent standard open surgery in US [15]. On the other hand open thoracic aorta prosthetic substitution still carries significant risk of serious complications that cannot be fully prevented even in very highly specialized centers, in particular to CNS and spinal cord.

Although the pathogenesis of these complications is multifactorial, there is general agreement that the length of clamping/circulatory arrest time is an extremely important factor. Since nearly all the clamping/arrest time is spent for vascular anastomosis construction, a device able to quicken and simplify the vascular anastomosis can be expected to have a significant impact on the incidence of these complications.

Suture line haemostasis is also an important source of intra- and postoperative complications with standard open technique. In fact due to the altered aortic wall mechanical features, impaired by the underlying aortic pathology (arteriosclerosis, medial cystic degeneration, Marfan syndrome etc.), the suture line haemostasis may be difficult to achieve in spite of appropriate surgical technique or may require additional surgical maneuvers (buttressing, gluing etc.) that imply prolongation of the ischemia time.

Moreover in cases of dissection, it may be difficult to achieve firm layers approximation and to prevent re-dissection and false lumen persistent perfusion, in particular at suture lines.

For these reasons several years ago we started research [25] to develop a new expandable device aimed: 1-to simplify the surgical technique; 2-to significantly reduce the ischemic time and thus the ischemic complications rate; 3-to enhance suture line anastomosis; 4-to achieve firm and reliable dissected layers approximation, thus preventing re-dissection and/or false lumen persistent perfusion at suture lines, particularly in acute dissection repairs.

The device consists of loops of nitinol wires, wrapped within a Dacron fabric and connected to a prosthesis end (Type I and III). The nitinol wire loops can be expanded and tightened by activating a removable guide in such a way that device end varies its diameter, while maintaining a regular cylindrical shape (Figure 9). This allows the easy and quick insertion of the retracted device into the vascular stump and then its expansion to perfectly fit with the vessel diameter; haemostasis and permanent device fixation is provided by external ligature/suture.

It's quite evident that the expandable configuration of the ring (Figure 10) allows to solve all the insertion, positioning and stability problems of the 70ies intraluminal prosthesis. That makes performing an anastomosis a very simple task, which can be carried out in seconds vs. the 10-15 min per anastomosis at best required with standard hand suture. The aortic wall being not perforated by the suture all around, the coupling is immediately blood-thigh ("air-tight" in fact!) and then independent by the integrity of the physiological coagulation mechanisms.

The device underwent many modifications and refinements, finally resulting in three main models (Type I, II and III) applying the same working mechanism, but with different shape to fit with all aorta segments as well as special conditions of use.

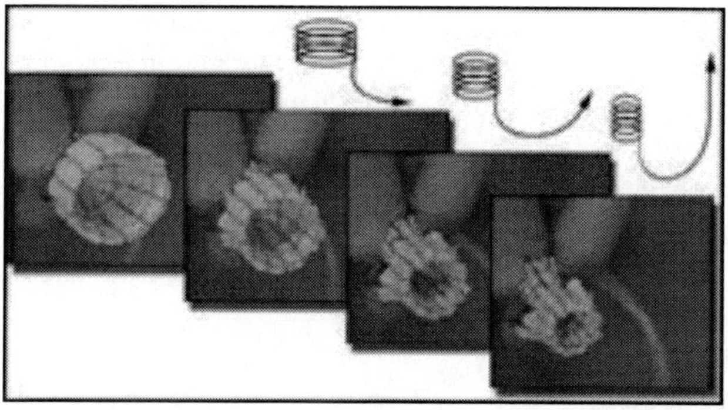

Figure 9. Expandable device working principle. Loops of nitinol wire wrapped by Dacron fabric form a rigid sleeve whose diameter can be modified by varying the diameter of the nitinol loops, while the regular cylindrical shape is maintained (from 26 with permission).

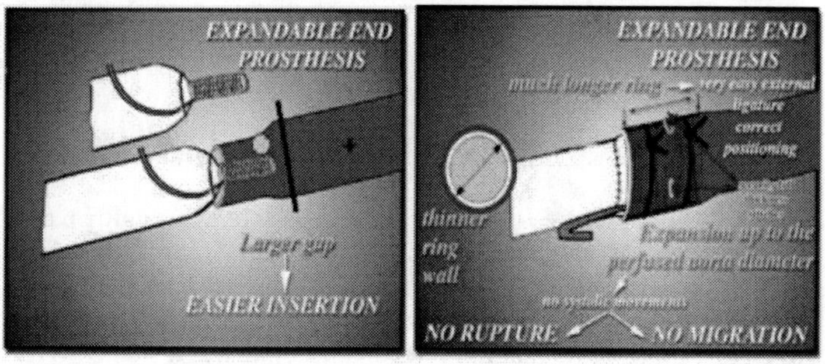

Figure 10. Expandable device vs. intraluminal ringed prosthesis. The expandable configuration of the ring allows to solve all the insertion, positioning and diameter mismatch problems of the 70ies intraluminal prosthesis.

Extensive "ex vivo" and "in vivo" animal experiments [25-28, 30, 31, 32, 36] were carried out and few clinical cases were also successfully treated with this device [29, 1, 5].

2.1. Device Description and Operational Details

2.1.1. Device Type I and II

Device type I and II differ because of the orientation of the activating guide in respect to the main axis of the device wireframe expandable sleeve (Figure 11); that allows the devices to be ideally used for the first and second anastomosis respectively.

Thus the type I device, sutured at one end of the tube graft of appropriate size before clamping, is activated by guide-wire coaxial to the lumen and then can be quickly and easily positioned into the vascular stump of the first anastomosis, either in the proximal or distal end of the aortic tract to be replaced (Figure 12 upper squares row). Appropriate device aperture is then temporarily blocked by bending up to 60-90 degree the proximal end of the activating guide (Figure 12, white outlined smaller squares) order to prevent nitinol wire, laying in stainless steel tube in this tract, from sliding backwards and tourniquet tightened.

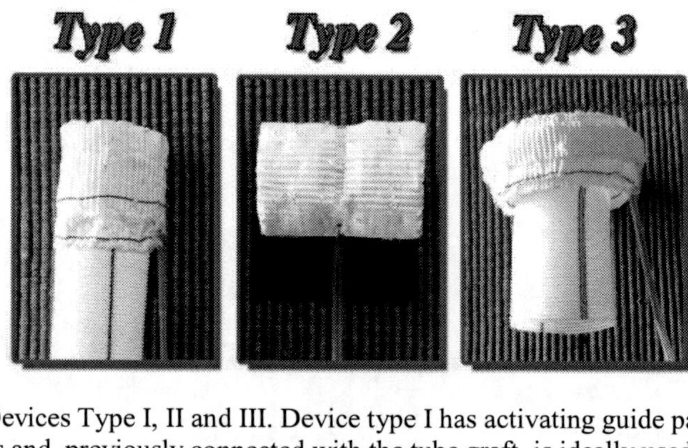

Figure 11. Devices Type I, II and III. Device type I has activating guide parallel to the vascular axis and, previously connected with the tube graft, is ideally used for the first anastomosis either proximal or distal. In device type II the activating guide perpendicular to the vascular axis divides the expandable sleeve in two segments for connecting the two stumps of ideally the second anastomosis. Device type III incorporates an external sleeve that substitutes the external ligature, thus allowing full control of the pressure applied to the vascular stump, useful in particular condition of fragility of the aortic wall as acute dissection.

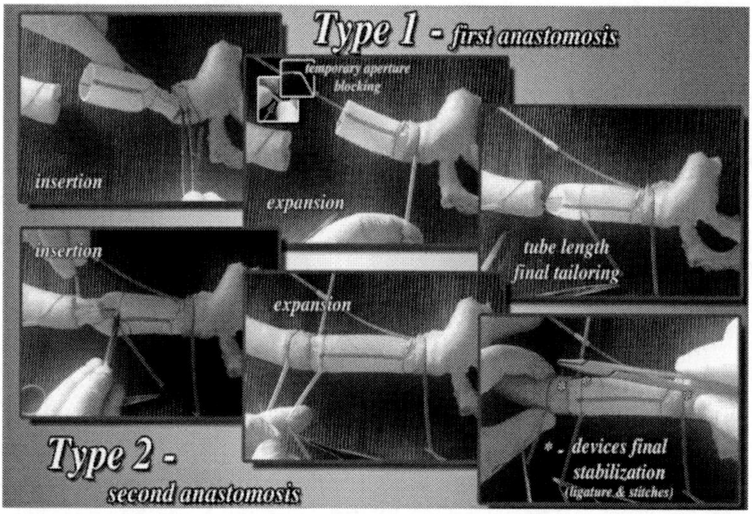

Figure 12. Devices type I and II in "ex vivo" descending aorta swine model. Upper strip: Device type I, previously sutured to the appropriate diameter tube graft end, is used for the first anastomosis, either proximal or distal; its aperture is temporarily fixed by bending up to 60-90 degree the proximal end of the activating guide (small white outlined squares). Then after having carried out any other collateral branch anastomosis possibly required, the tube graft is cut at its appropriate final measure and fixed with a single stitch at rear anastomosis side Lower strip: device Type II is applied for the anastomosis and aperture temporarily fixed. Circulation can be immediately resumed after tourniquets tightening. Final ligature (haemostasis), full thickness stitches (stabilization) at each anastomosis and activating guides removal (figure 14) can be then carried out without prolonging the ischemic phase.

Any further manipulation of the tube graft is then easily possible, including accessory side anastomosis with aortic branches, without any hindrance.

The tube graft can then be sectioned at its exact required length and fixed with a single stitch at the rear anastomosis side (Figure 12, upper row, right square). Type II device, activated by guide-wire orthogonal to the vascular axis allowing stump connection at both sides, is then inserted, expanded, expansion temporarily blocked by folding the distal end of the activating guide and haemostasis immediately achieved by tourniquets retraction at both stumps (Figure 12, lower row, middle square) thus ending the ischemia phase.

After having resumed the circulation, the permanent fixation of each of the three stumps (Figure 12, * at lower row, right square) is carried out by tying ligature (haemostasis) and applying two or three full thickness polypropylene 4-0 approximately equidistant stitches (stabilization), virtually preventing any possible late dislocation. Use tourniquets (umbilical tape or polypropylene) obviously minimizes the ischemic time, allowing to carry out the final stabilization on the perfused stumps. In particular circumstances when full stump isolations could be better avoided, polypropylene suture can be passed, totally or partially, from inside the vascular lumen in a purse-string fashion with the same haemostatic results (Figure 13). It is however important to complete the fixation by passing the suture full thickness through the device at least in 2-3 roughly equidistant points in order to prevent any possible late dislocation.

Immediately after appropriate expandable end positioning and expansion, the temporary aperture blockage is achieved by simple bending up to 60-90 degree the distal end of the activating guide; that in fact prevents nitinol wire, laying in stainless steel tube in this tract, from sliding backwards and then from modification of aperture and otherwise possible displacement (Figure 14 A). When the blood flow is re-established the final fixation is achieve by bending up to 180 degree the activating guide as close as possible to the expandable end and kept in that position be a ligature; the distal guide is then sectioned (Figure14 B, red arrows) and removed.

Few technical details must be considered when using expandable devices.

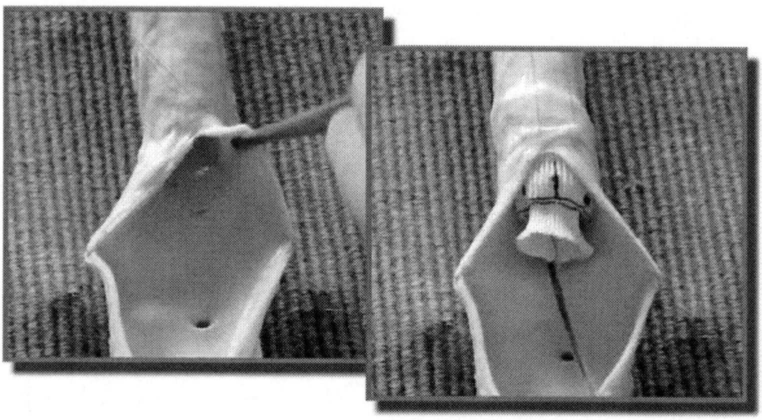

Figure 13. Device ligature from inside. If opportune, the vascular stump encirclement can be avoided and substituted by endovascular (full or partial) purse-string like polypropylene suture previously prepared at the site of expandable device positioning. The required full thickness security stitches can be passed after the circulation has been re-established (from 32, with permission).

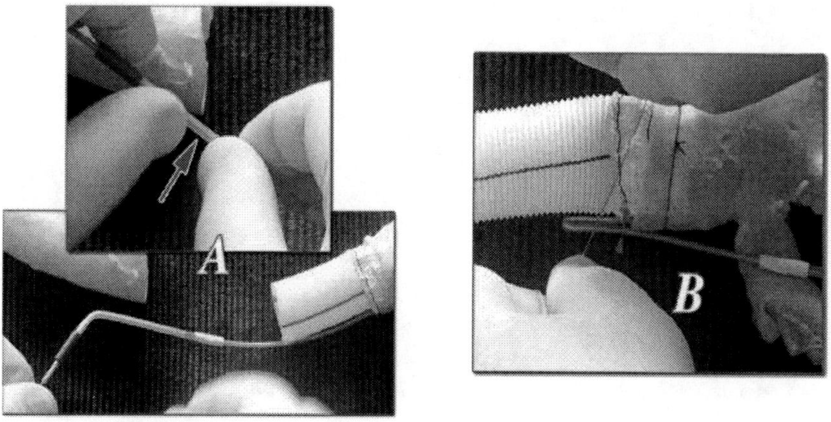

Figure 14. Temporary fixation and final guide removal. Temporary fixation is obtained by bending the distal end of the activating guide (A). After circulation is re-established the guide is bended up to 180 degree, fixed by ligature and cut away (B, red arrows).

First of all care must be taken when entering the aneurysm not to extend the incision up to both the distal and proximal ends as usually carried out with standard suture; it is in fact important to keep intact the entire circumference of the vascular stump for a tract long enough to host the device expandable end.

Due to the linearization of the vessel diameter induced by the clamp, the length of the vascular stump distal to it must be significantly longer than imagined before clamping; in practice it is advisable to isolate the vessel for a length exceeding its diameter (Figure 15, left square).

It may be argued that the use of the device may require a distinct healthy vascular neck, as with endovascular techniques. That is not necessary. The device in fact can be expanded even within the aneurismal wall and fixed there by the external ligature and stitches, provided that its end reaches the healthy vascular wall limit, where ideally the standard suture would be placed (Figure 15, right square).

The thrombosis developing in the tract between the ligature and the prosthesis end will soon exclude the brief tract of aneurismal wall from the bloodstream, thus moving the effective anastomosis line (Figure 15,* at upper right square) where it would be with standard suture.

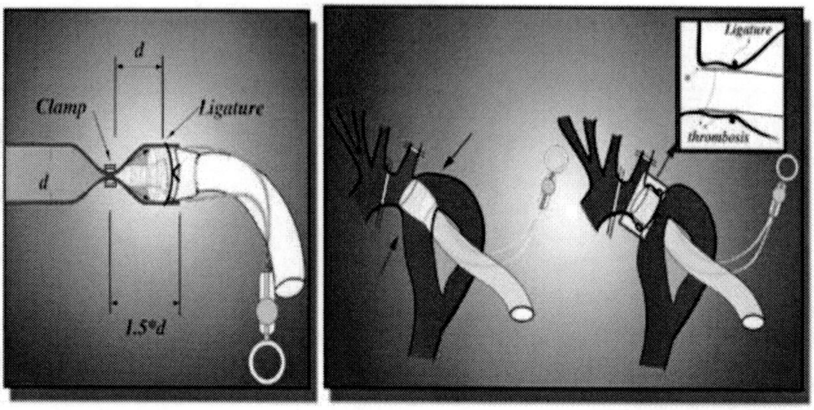

Figure 15. Expandable device operational details. Left square: When a clamp is applied the linearization of the stump requires to keep its length significantly longer than usual in order to leave the space necessary for full expansion of the expandable end. It is also important to avoid full longitudinal vascular opening as carried out with current technique and thus keeping intact the entire circumference of the vascular stump for a tract long enough to host the whole device expandable end. Right square: The expandable end also can be positioned against aneurismal wall, provided that its distal end would reach the healthy vascular wall. Thrombosis of the tract between the ligature and the prosthesis end will soon move the effective anastomosis line (upper right square*) where it would be with standard suture (mod from 28 with permission).

Thus devices type I and II can be ideally used anywhere in descending thoracic and abdominal aorta and allow to carry out any required additional surgical maneuver on the tube graft, i.e. collateral branch anastomosis, as well as its appropriate tailoring at the required length measured directly on the operative field as in standard technique without obstacles or hampering conditions. Its great simplicity of use allows the devices to be used also in condition of suboptimal operative field exposure. Thus for example both proximal and distal anastomosis in extended descending thoracic aorta substitution can be easily and safely carried out though a single space thoracotomy; moreover aortic prosthetic substitution via mini-access thoracotomy or laparotomy video-assisted setting may be also predictably possible and certainly more easy than standard suture technique.

2.1.2. Device Type III

In this version of the device the external ligature is substituted by an expandable sleeve, which is based essentially on the same working principle as the inner sleeve, but activated contrariwise. Thus, the vascular stump is compressed between two sleeves (Figure 16, upper left little squares), with variable and controllable diameters, allowing full control of the pressure (amount and surface of its application) actually applied to the vascular stump.

Operative technique for device type III is illustrated in Figure 16 in ascending aorta swine "ex vivo" model and it is really very simple. First of all both sleeves diameter is set at the predicted value of the aortic tract where the device will be applied. Then by acting on its guide-wire the inner sleeve only its diameter is reduced as much as an easy insertion into the vascular stump is possible; the inner sleeve diameter reduction causes also the backwards rotation and eversion of the outer sleeve thus greatly enhancing inner sleeve visibility and then its easy positioning into the vascular stump. The inner sleeve is then re-expanded against the vascular stump inner surface; at this point the outer sleeve is gently retracted acting on its own activating guide to compress the vascular stump. Temporary and final aperture of inner and outer sleeves as well as guide removal is carried out with the same technique indicated for type I and II devices at Figure 14.

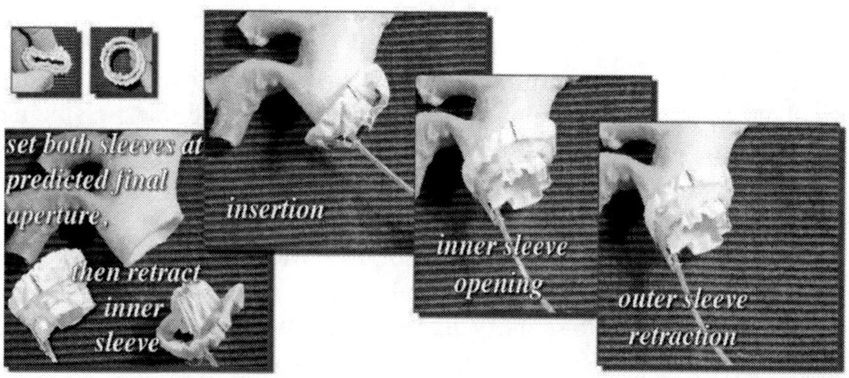

Figure 16. Device type III. The wire-frame of the device is quite soft and compliant, and can be easily compressed and widely deformed while maintaining perfect reciprocal alignment of the internal and external sleeves (top left squares) and is intended ideally for use in dissection cases or when the aortic wall may need some form of buttressing. Lower squares: "ex vivo" ascending aorta swine model. First of all both sleeves are set at predicted final aperture. The acting on the activating guide of the inner sleeve only results in the backwards rotation and eversion of the outer sleeve, bringing the retracted inner sleeve in full visibility, so that it can be easily inserted into the vascular stump. Then inner ring is then expanded so that the vascular wall is pushed against the outer sleeve inner surface. At this point, the outer sleeve is only slightly retracted towards the aortic wall using its own guide. Temporary and final aperture stabilization and guide removal is carried out in the same way as with type 1 or II devices (figure 14). Video at http://www.fondazionecarrel.org/nazarichaptervideo.html.

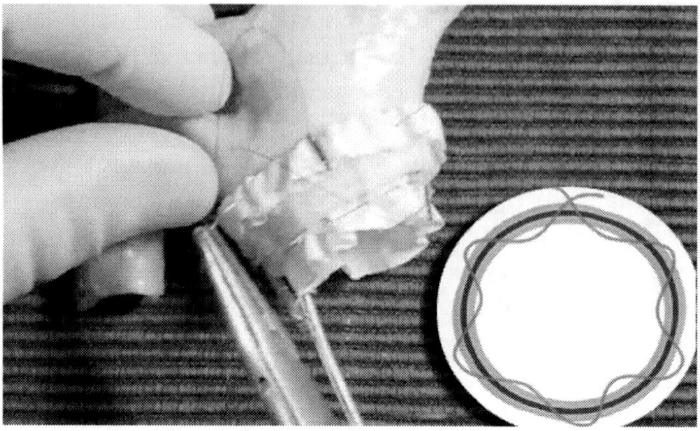

Figure 17. Type III security fixation. A simple in and out 3 or 4-0 prolene in several points linking the inner and outer device wireframe and aortic stump will greatly increase coupling stability and can be carried out easily and quickly when circulation is resumed. Video at http://www.fondazionecarrel.org/nazarichaptervideo.html.

Even though needles present on the outer surface may be sufficient to provide stability when the aortic wall is compressed by the outer ring, we think that polypropylene 3 or 4 0 running suture with several full thickness, in and out, circumferential passages firmly linking aortic stump with inner and outer expandable sleeves (Figure 17) may add absolute safety in an easy and quick way that may be carried out when circulation is resumed.

The primary aim of this new version of the device is to make possible and convenient to apply this coupling principle also to acute ascending aorta and arch dissection, in order to simplify the technique, to reduce the ischemic time, to improve hemostasis of the anastomosis line and to achieve reliable, stable sealing of the dissection layers in this very complex surgical setting.

Type III device in fact allows to actually automate substantially the same aortic wall sandwiching between two graft strips procedure usually carried out in the dissection cases and to realize at once the tube prosthesis anastomosis, being the tube graft (not shown in the figure 16) obviously previously sutured to the inner sleeve. Interestingly enough the particular configuration of the device allows full and easy compliance with aortic anatomy, perfectly adapting also to the elliptic, asymmetric "oblique" stump resulting from inclusion of the arch concavity in the anastomosis line.

In fact full and persistent air-tight sealing of the device-aortic wall coupling was verified at endovascular pressures of up to 150 mmHg in "ex vivo" swine aortic models, including those involving an elliptic, 'oblique' anastomosis (Figure 18, b) [32]. Interestingly enough standard vascular sutures were not "air-tight" even at pressures below 10 mmHg (Figure 18, c).

The solution of positioning and stability problems of the 70ies intraluminal prosthesis (Figure 10) allows for the first time the clinical appreciation of the most important feature of the "Payr principle" of anastomosis (vascular stumps compression against/between rigid structures i.e. an inner rigid ring and external ligature/outer rigid ring) which is to achieve an immediate hermetic seal ("air-tight" in fact) ensuring reliable haemostasis at the anastomosis line, not dependent from coagulation. Interestingly enough were just the positioning problems of Payr model as well as of its more recent modification (intraluminal ringed prosthesis), that prevented the clinical implementation of this coupling method, which is the most intuitive (and in fact was the first to be attempted even in vascular surgery) and whose application failed only in the surgical field, while was in use, and still is, in all other technological fields where connectors between elastic/floppy tubing are required.

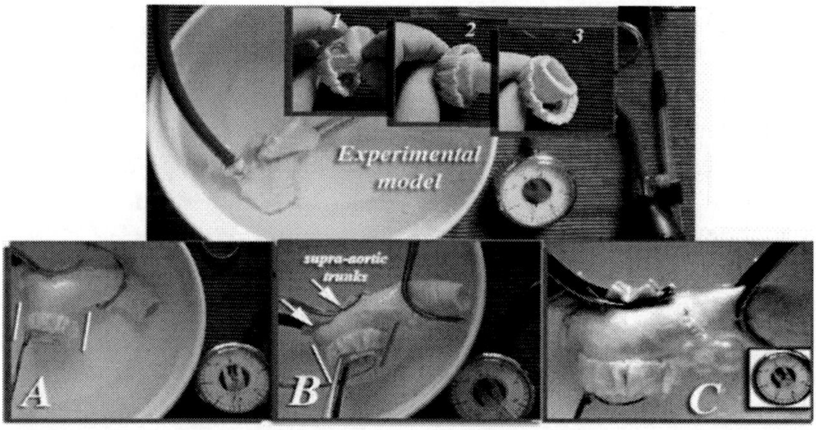

Figure 18. Device type III seal test. The outer surface of the inner sleeve was wrapped by a latex cuff (top squares) in order to overcome the problem of the porosity of the Dacron graft and the requirement for the connection of the tube graft to the proximal end of the inner sleeve as in its final clinical use. A) The air-tightness of the connection was verified at endovascular pressures of up to 150 mmHg in a regular cylindrical anastomosis of ascending aorta (white bars). (B) The same was verified when the anastomosis is irregularly oriented, such as when involves the arch concavity. (C) As easily predictable, a standard suture (4–0 prolene) of an approximately 3 cm incision of the aortic wall cannot be proved airtight even at minor endovascular pressure (modify. from 32 with permission). Video at http://www.fondazionecarrel.org/ nazarichaptervideo.html.

Of course clinical experience over more than a century has shown that the standard suturing technique does not need to provide an "air-tight" anastomosis to ensure perfect hemostasis in virtually all clinical circumstances. In particular cases however (acute dissection, Marfan [16] and other genetic disorders, cystic medial necrosis, etc.), structural impairments of the aortic wall may necessitate additional maneuvers including graft strips buttressing, gluing and a variety of accessory techniques, whose efficacy at achieving haemostasis are not always fully predictable and that obviously further significantly prolong the period of ischemia in this most critical area. A coupling method that provides haemostasis by compression of the stumps' vascular wall between two rigid structures (i.e. inner and outer expandable rigid sleeves) without perforation may be then particularly useful in these cases, not only because of its ease and quickness, but also because it offers the best mechanical chance of immediate blood-tightness. The expected advantages with regards to approximation of dissecting layers and false lumen permanent sealing rely on the same mechanical concept.

Another important difference with 70-80ies intraluminal ringed devices is that the expandable sleeve is much more thin and porous, being formed substantially by a double layer of standard vascular Dacron fabric, and can, therefore, be wholly and quickly colonized by fibroblasts and soon integrated within the aortic wall. The nitinol wire-frame in fact forms a very thin and wide mesh net that accounts only for a very small proportion of the device's volume and that offers no significant barrier to fibroblastic invasion of the Dacron fabric and thus to stable biological integration of the device.

Type III device use can be then ideally indicated in dissection cases for distal anastomosis sited at distal ascending aorta, including as much as required of the concavity of the arch during a very brief circulatory arrest phase; proximal anastomosis will be then carried out either by hand suture or with the expandable device version most appropriated for the particular anatomical condition, in normal CEC in no rush and after having performed any additional procedure possibly required, for example on the valve.

Anastomosis at the distal arch/proximal descending aorta in case of full arch substitution is also an ideal indication for type III device use in case of dissection or whenever, for particular aortic wall fragility, graft strips sandwiching buttressing may be advisable. Thus in all cases where sandwiching buttressing is planned, the use of the device type III requires exactly the same aortic stump external wall preparation required for hand suture double graft strips application with the advantage of realizing it much more quickly and at once with the tube graft anastomosis.

When compared with device I or II the double ring configuration of device type III allows a very significant reduction of its length, thus greatly enhance its positioning into the curved anatomy of the ascending aorta and arch without any orientation conflict, even allowing an asymmetric disposition of the expandable sleeves in different area of the anastomosis without losing "air-tight" competence.

The great simplification and the very significant quickening of this complex surgical part together with the higher accuracy and "mechanical" reliability of this coupling method in comparison with manual suture could potentially have impact that may exceed that strictly related to the anastomosis. For example being possible to carry out even the entire arch re-vascularization in very few minutes of circulatory arrest, the level of hypothermia may be significantly reduced and even the type of cerebral protection may be tailored to these very restricted time lapses, when supraortic trunks anstomosis is carried out by graft assembled with appropriate devices' combination (see below), just to say the firsts coming in mind.

2.2. Other Expandable Device Models and Combinations

We also realized a variety of modified versions of the device to better fit with the anatomical configurations occurring in particular clinical circumstances.

2.2.1. Type I with Single Outer Layer for Small Diameters

In small vessel diameters device fabric wrapping can interfere more significantly with effective lumen amplitude in their range of use. More in particular the way of folding of the inner fabric layer when the device is incompletely opened may reduce the lumen effectively available for the blood flow to an extent that may be difficult to predict. Accordingly for diameters $\leq$ 12 and $\geq$6 mm we prepared devices wrapped by un-crimped thin fabric positioned only at external side of the nitinol wireframe. Three sizes were prepared respectively for diameter from 6-8 mm, 8-10 and from 10 to 12 mm. The device is previously prepared at the end of collateral branch of the main tube graft cut at the expected appropriated length or directly on the main tube graft (see Figure 20, 21, 22 and 23). The ideal evolution of this project however would probably consider devices size appropriate to each currently available small diameter tube graft size, mounted at an un-crimped part of one of its end.

This device type may ideally fit for renal, celiac, mesenteric art. and supraortic trunks as well as for any vessel with diameter $\geq$ 6 mm.

2.2.2. Type II Bendable and with Independent Opening

This type II device modified version is intended for use in ascending aorta substitution in absence of dissection. The two ends of the device can vary their reciprocal axis up to 90° to better fit with the curvature of the ascending aorta; their aperture can be independently controlled in order to comply with possible differences in diameter of the proximal and distal stumps (Figure 19). In this way the ascending aorta substitution in anatomically suitable cases can be carried out very quickly by one single device.

In case of dissection however type III device previously connected with graft tube should be better used at distal or both anastomosis. Various possible combinations between device types can ideally fit any particular anatomical occurrence. Anyway proximal anastomosis can be carried out with standard suture, time being not here a critical factor, or by a second type III device if suggested by the quality of the proximal vascular stump.

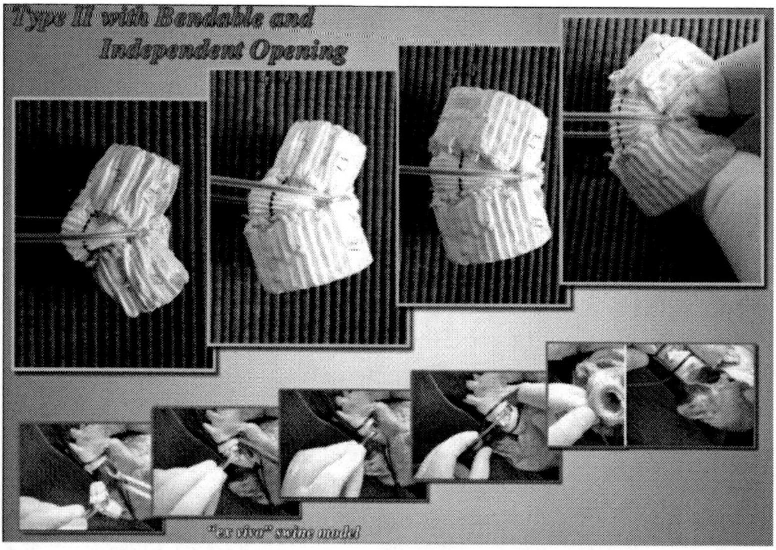

Figure 19. Device Type II Bendable and with Independent Opening. This type II device version allows the bending up to a 90° degree angle of the axis of their ends, whose aperture can be independently controlled. This allows to fit curved anatomy of ascending aorta and possible variations in diameter of the vascular stumps. The lower strip shows the device application in "ex-vivo" swine ascending aorta model. Video at: http://www.fondazionecarrel.org/nazarichaptervideo.html.

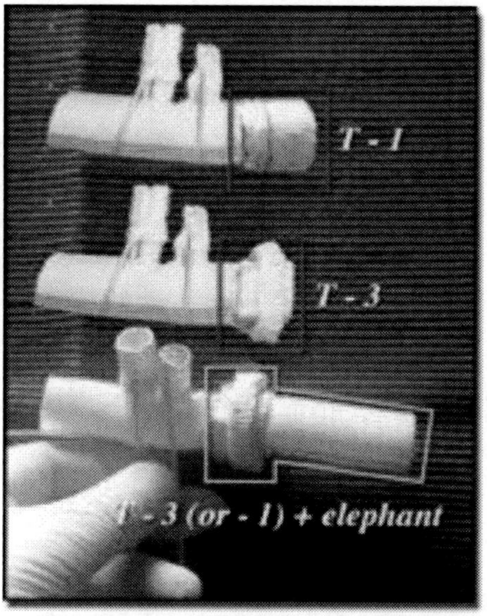

Figure 20. Composite configuration for arch substitution (swine model). Distal anastomosis is performed with type I or 3 devices according to the presence of dissection or poor quality of aortic stump as well as distal aorta pathology; in case type I is used full isolation of the distal anastomosis site can be as usually avoided and device fixed by passing the ligature, totally or only in part from inside as shown in figure 11. Type I devices with single outer layer is used if the supraortic trunk inner diameter is less then 12 mm. The illustrated prototypes are shaped to fit with "ex vivo" swine anatomy.

This device version can also be ideally suitable for isthmus rupture repair, having care of entering the aorta through or close to the laceration in order to preserve integrity of the vascular wall at site of device ends deployment; obviously the left subclavian artery origin may not allow room for proximal device deployment and then re-implant or by-pass can be considered if deemed advantageous in time critical conditions.

2.2.3. Composite Configurations

2.2.3.1. Aortic Arch

With expandable devices appropriately prepared on tube graft it is possible to quickly connect supra-aortic trunks and proximal descending aorta during a very short circulatory arrest phase. The ideal configuration of tube graft include expandable device at its distal end for distal arch-proximal descending aorta anastomosis, the type being selected on the basis of vascular stump and descending aorta conditions (Figure 20). Moreover type I devices appropriate to supraortic trunks size (single outer layer for inner diameters ≤ 12 mm) are previously prepared ideally on branched tube graft whose length is tailored according to the occurring anatomy before circulatory arrest. Elephant trunk (original or frozen) procedure is also easily performed also when type III device is to be used for distal arch anastomosis, here illustrated in "ex vivo" swine anatomy compatible prototypes (Figure 21); in fact backwards displacement of the outer sleeve when the inner one is retracted greatly enhance insertion of the elephant trunk and appropriate vascular stump positioning to be compressed between the device's sleeves whose final aperture can be adjusted to the most appropriate diameter. The particular configuration of prototypes for human anatomy and size suitable for aortic arch substitution (Figure 22) allows an easy and effective compensation of even wide discrepancy between aortic diameter and elephant trunk.

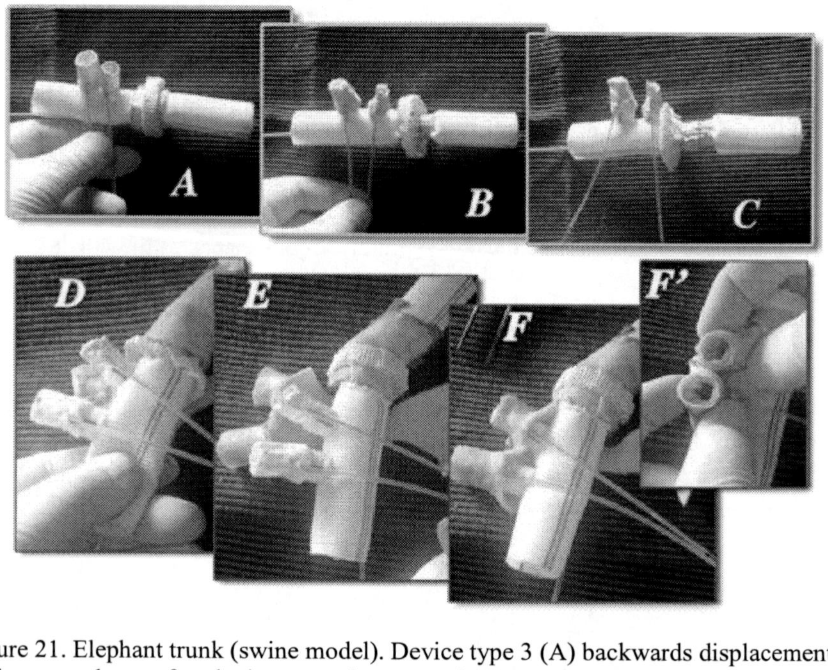

Figure 21. Elephant trunk (swine model). Device type 3 (A) backwards displacement of the outer sleeve after the inner one is retracted (C) greatly enhance insertion of the elephant trunk and appropriate vascular stump positioning (D) to be compressed between the device's sleeves (E); the easy and quick supraortic trunks is then carried out (F,F') Video at: http://www.fondazionecarrel.org/nazarichaptervideo.html.

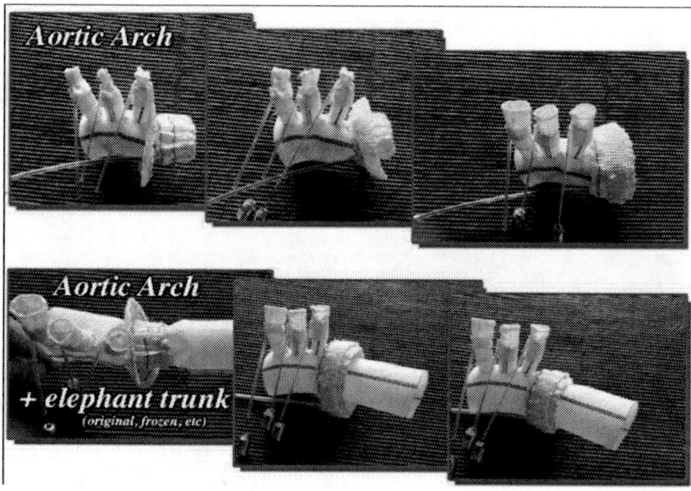

Figure 22. Human configuration prototypes for aortic arch. Figure illustrates prototypes human anatomy and size (outer sleeve 55 mm, tube graft 36 mm) suitable for arch substitution.

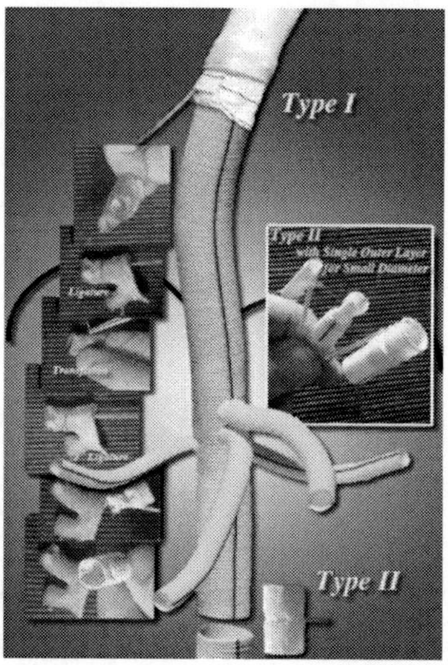

Figure 23. Thoraco-abdominal Aorta. Expandable device type I, ≧6 mm in diameter, with single outer Dacron layer (red squares) can be prepared on appropriately tailored branches of Coselli's type tube graft for quick connections of main visceral aortic collaterals. This version of device type I for small diameters was prepared with single outer un-crimped fabric graft in order to prevent the possible significant interference with vascular lumen of unpredictable way of folding of the inner layer when the device cannot be fully expanded.

2.2.3.2. Thoraco-Abdominal Aorta

Type I devices with graft single outer layer as small as 6 mm in diameter can also be previously prepared on branches of Coselli's tube (Figure 23) tailored in length appropriated to the patient anatomy before clamping allowing; this can significantly simplify and quickening this still very critical clinical condition.

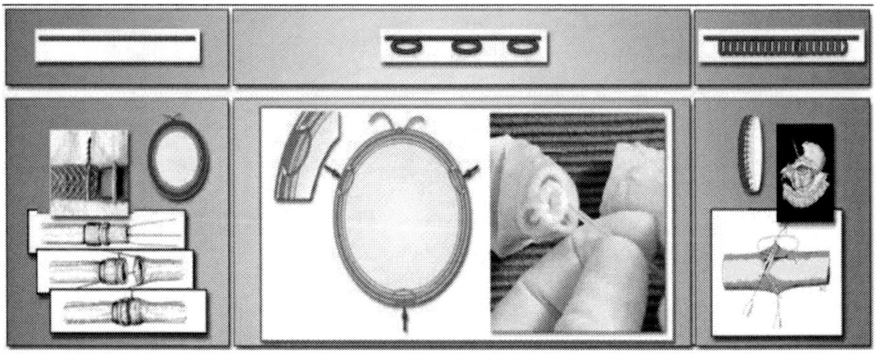

Figure 24. External ligature and scattered transfixion - a meeting point. Reliable coupling stability, instead of simple external ligature is achieved by few prolene 3-0 or 4-0 encircling suture, transfixing full thickness the device and aortic wall stump at few (2 or more approximately equidistant) points, passed and tied as shown. It may be then speculate that expandable configuration of the prosthesis end made possible a quite advantageous meeting point between the first endeavor (Payr) and current technique (Carrel) for vascular-graft anastomosis. Video at http://www.fondazionecarrel.org/nazarichaptervideo.html.

Conclusion and Perspectives

The extensive past experience provided full mechanical reliability of devices in all their versions and proved their easy applicability to aortic stump in all conditions in "ex vivo" models. Animal experience and successful clinical application in few clinical case confirmed that expandable devices provide very significant advantages over current hand suture anastomosis in aortic prosthetic substitution.

While the expandable device allows a much easier, quicker and more efficient ("airtight" seal) graft-aortic stump coupling than standard suture [32], it may be argued however that the permanence of endovascular tubular wireframe and external ligature could, in particular circumstances, mechanically conflict with aortic wall, particularly at device ends, and/or with confining tissues/organs.

Aorto-digestive fistula is an infrequent but well documented occurrence after aortic open [14, 22] as well as after endovascular [37, 23, 10] repair. While graft or/and suture line contamination/infection may occasionally be suspected as the primary etiological factor, pure mechanical erosion from systolic or other causes movements of graft and even from the suture line only [40] may probably represent the first triggering factor in a fraction of cases difficult to quantify. The pure mechanical effect of these movements on the confining tissue/organ is predictably higher the harder/less compliant is the prosthetic material as well as the more conflicting is its orientation in relation to the confining tissue/organ. We then recently focused on optimal consistency of the expandable wireframe and on means to provide external fixation with the final aim of achieving mechanical forces of coupling as much as possible similar to those taking place in standard hand suture anastomosis.

For this purpose, on one side, the wireframe consistency was decreased by variably reducing the gauge of nitinol wires and their respective position within wireframe and, on the other side, the external ligature was carried out with the thinnest possible prolene (4-0 / 5-0) encircling suture, transfixing full thickness the device and aortic wall at two or three approximately equidistant points. The mechanical limit of the former was the ability to sustain the external ligature without wireframe deformation/collapse at pressure providing "airtight" seal; the limit of the later was the ability to provide stability of the aortic stump-expandable device coupling at stretch test.

The present versions of the devices minimize the risk of mechanical conflict and erosion with the confining tissue/organs; moreover wireframe consistency was settled in such a way that is minimal (thinner nitinol wire) at the device distal end where the possible conflict with aortic wall could be higher. However a tighter surgical limit to reduction of nitinol wire diameter and then overall wireframe consistency is related to the necessity to preserve the ability of the device to actively expand the vascular stump enough to achieve the expected diameter when blood perfusion is resumed. Ex-vivo experiments showed that this goal requires nitinol wire diameters significantly greater than those required for simple achieving haemostasis and stability by external ligature.

Moreover the variable conditions of vascular stump may also suggest in this regard different devices wireframe consistency ranging from the lowest, appropriate for example in case of dissection, to the strongest in presence of heavy calcification/atherosclerosis. Accordingly it seems important to provide each device type and version in two or three different wireframe consistencies (i.e. strong, standard, light) to adequately fit with all clinical conditions.

Concerning the external ligature and its many possible ways of application, it may be useful to recall again that haemostatic seal and stability of the expandable device anastomosis, contrariwise to standard suture, rely on different mechanisms (Figure 8).

Thus even though external devices surface is provided with short needles perpendicularly positioned around its circumference at 4-6 equidistant points, reduction of the wireframe consistency may probably decrease their reliability in keeping coupling stability. We then think that it is very important to optimize coupling stability adding to the external ligature, transfixing full thickness the device and aortic wall at least in two or three approximately equidistant points.

The stability of this coupling in its many possible variations was checked by a stretch test model consisting in a sequence of maneuvers carried out on the anastomosis that includes: 1) complete compression of the anastomosis in orthogonal directions and then 2) vigorous manual stretching of the anastomosis in the coaxial plane separately at four points of its circumference. The sequence was repeated three times and the anastomosis checked for any significant vascular stump backwards dislocation on the expandable wireframe throughout the entire circumference (Video at: http://www.fondazionecarrel.org/nazarichaptervideo.html).

This allowed to refine details involved in this procedure (external ligature + 2/3 stitches fixation) that can be ideally carried out with polypropylene suture, 3 to 5-0 depending on the vascular stump consistency and diameter, positioned either in two steps, i.e. encircling ligature and vascular wall-device transfixion stitches or with a single step the suture being passed in the way indicated in Figure 23.

Device type III stability is also increased by further buttressing the inner and outer Dacron wrapping by 4-0 prolene suture transfixing the circumference in several points (Figure 17). In synthesis this method ideally allows to convert any vascular-graft anastomosis $\geq$ 6 mm in diameter from the current facing ends Carrel suture into a simpler, quicker and more efficient ("airtight" seal) telescoping anastomosis, sealed and fixed by single thread external ligature passed full thickness at two/three points (or more when appropriate), in a sort of ideal optimized meeting point between Payr first and Carrel current technique.

Table 1. Potential impact of expandable device aortic anastomosis compared with current hand suture technique

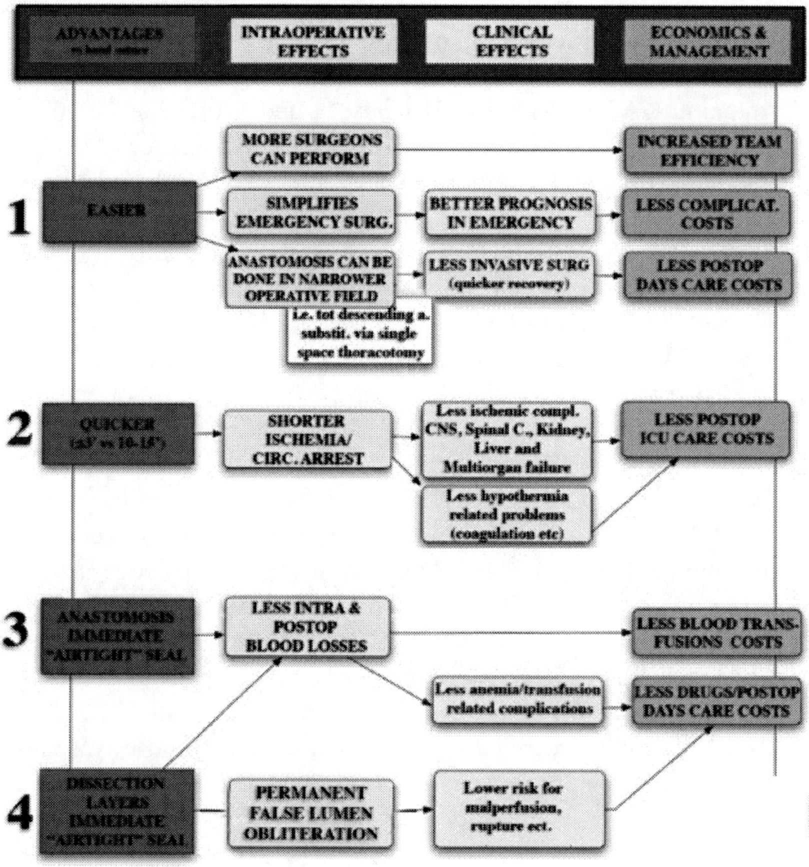

The hypothesizable potential impact (table 1) may exceed that expected on complication rate of open prosthetic substitution of all aortic tracts and in particular in those higher risk conditions as acute dissection.

In fact the technical simplification with increased reliability of anastomosis haemostasis and dissection layer approximation with false lumen permanent seal has the logical direct consequence, for example, of enabling also lesser expert cardiovascular surgeons to deal with these clinical cases very often requiring immediate surgical attention, thus increasing surgical team efficiency and hospital unit productivity.

References

[1] Aluffi A, Buniva P, Rescigno G and Nazari S. (2002) Improved device for sutureless aortic anastomosis applied in a case of cancer. *Tex. Heart Inst. J.* 29: 56–59.

[2] Antoniou GA, El Sakka K, Hamady M and Wolfe JH. (2010) Hybrid treatment of complex aortic arch disease with supraaortic debranching and endovascular stent graft repair. *Eur. J. Vasc. Endovasc. Surg.* 39:683-90.

[3] Berger RL, Romero L, Chaudhry AG and Dobnik DB.(1983) Graft replacement of the thoracic aorta with a sutureless technique. *Ann. Thorac. Surg.* 35:231–239.

[4] Brown LC, Thompson SG, Greenhalgh RM and Powell JT (2011): Incidence of cardiovascular events and death after open or endovascular repair of abdominal aortic aneurysm in the randomized EVAR trial 1. *British Journal of Surgery* 98: 935–942.

[5] Buniva P, Rescigno G, Salvi S, Aluffi A, Berti A. Salsi F, Nazari S (2002) Sutureless expandable end prosthesis for descending aorta substitution invaded by bronchogenic cancer. Video, *Proceedings Aortic Surgery Symposium VIII, New York,* May 2-3, 2002.

[6] Canaud L, Hireche K, Berthet JP et al.(2010): Endovascular repair of aortic arch lesions in high-risk patients or after previous aortic surgery: midterm results. *J. Thorac. Cardiovasc. Surg.* 140:52-8.

[7] Carrel A. (1902) La technique operatoire des anastomoses vasculaires et la transplantation des visceres. *Lyon Med.* 98:859–864.

[8] CarrelA. (1907) The surgery of blood vessels. *Bull. Johns Hopkins Hosp.;* 18: 18–27.

[9] Charnsangavej C, Wallace S, Wright KC, Carrasco CH and Gianturco C. (1985) Endovascular stent for use in aortic dissection: an in vitro experiment. *Radiology.*157:323-4.

[10] Chiesa R, Melissano G, Marone EM, Marrocco-Trischitta MM and Kahlberg A (2010)Aorto- oesophageal and aortobronchial fistulae following thoracic endovascular aortic repair: a national survey. *Eur. J. Vasc. Endovasc. Surg.* 39:273-9.

[11] Crawford ES and Crawford JL, editors (1984). *Diseases of the aorta.* Baltimore: Williams and Wilkins, 61–77.

[12] De Bruin JL, Baas AF, Buth J, Prinssen M, Verhoeven EL, Cuypers PW et al.; DREAM Study Group.(2010) Long-term outcome of open or

endovascular repair of abdominal aortic aneurysm. *N. Engl. J. Med.* 362: 1881–1889.

[13] Di Eusanio M, Armaro A, Di Marco L, Pacini D, Savini C, Martin Suarez S, Pilato E and Di Bartolomeo R (2011) Short- and midterm results after hybrid treatment of chronic aortic dissection with the frozen elephant trunk technique. *Eur. J. Cardiothorac. Surg.* 2011 Oct; 40(4): 875-80. doi: 10.1016/j.ejcts.2011.01.068. Epub 2011 Mar 5.

[14] Geraci G, Pisello F, Li Volsi F, Facella T, Platia L, Modica G and Sciume C (2008) Secondary aortoduodenal fistula. *World J. Gastroenterol.* 14:484-6.

[15] Gopaldas RR., Huh J, Dao TK, LeMaire SA, Chu D, Bakaeen FG and Coselli JS (2010) Superior nationwide outcomes of endovascular versus open repair for isolated descending thoracic aortic aneurysm in 11,669 patients. *J. Thorac. Cardiovasc. Surg.* 140:1001-10.

[16] Gott VL, Laschinger JC, Cameron DE, Dietz HC, Greene PS, Gillinov AM, Pyeritz RE, Alejo DE, Fleischer KJ, Anhalt GJ, Stone CD and McKusick VA:(1996) The Marfan syndrome and the cardiovascular surgeon. *Eur. J. Cardiothorac. Surg.* 10:149-158.

[17] Kawaharada N, Ito T, Koyanagi T, Harada R, et al. (2010) Spinal cord protection with selective spinal perfusion during descending thoracic and thoracoabdominal aortic surgery. *Interact. CardioVasc. Thorac. Surg.* 10:986-991.

[18] Kolesov VI, Kolesov EV, Gurevich IY and Leosko VA.(1970) Vasosuturing apparatuses in surgery of coronary arteries. *Med. Tekhnika* 6:24–8.

[19] Kolesov VI and Kolesov EV. (1991) Twenty years' results with internal thoracic artery- coronary artery anastomosis [letter]. *J. Thorac. Cardiovasc. Surg.* 101:360–1.

[20] Konstantinov I E. (2004): Vasilii I. Kolesov A Surgeon to Remember. *Tex. Heart Inst. J.* 31: 349–358.

[21] Lemole GM, Strong MD, Spagna PM and Karilomicz MD (1982). Improved results for dissecting aneurysms: intraluminal sutureless prosthesis. J. Thorac. Cardiovasc. Surg. 83:249–255.

[22] Luo CY, Lai CH, Wen JS and Lin BW (2010) Secondary aortocolic fistula: case report and review of the literature. *Ann. Vasc. Surg.* 24: 256.e5-12.

[23] Marone EM, Esposito G, Kahlberg A, Tshomba Y, Brioschi C, Zannini P and Chiesa R. (2007) Surgical treatment of tracheoinnominate fistula

after stent- graft implantation. *J. Thorac. CardioVasc. Surg.* 133:1641–1643.

[24] Nazari S, Manelli A, Gastaldo A, Rinaldo A, Barana L and Zonta A. (1990) A new vascular stapler for pulmonary artery anastomosis in experimental single lung transplantation. Video, *Proceedings of the 4th Annual Meeting of the Association for Cardio-Thoracic Surgery,* Naples, September 16–19, 1990.

[25] Nazari S., Mourad Z, Luzzana F. (1994) Prosthetic substitution of the descending aorta without blood flow interruption. *Proceedings of the IV Aortic Surgery Symposium*, New York, April 20-22, 1994.

[26] Nazari S, Luzzana F, Banfi C, Mourad Z, Salvi S, Gaspari A and Nazari-Coerezza F.(1996) Expandable prosthesis for sutureless anastomosis in thoracic aorta prosthetic substitution. *Eur. J. Cardiothorac. Surg.* 10: 1003– 1009.

[27] Nazari S, Mourad Z, Banfi C, Salvi S, Visconti E, Aluffi A. (1996) Composite graft with expandable ends for total arch replacement. Video and Poster, *Proceedings Aortic Surgery Symposium* V, New York, April 23-26, 1996.

[28] Nazari S, Salvi S, Aluffi A, Visconti E, Rescigno G and Buniva P (1997) A new prosthesis for aortic arch substitution. *Ann. Thorac. Surg.* 64: 1339–1344.

[29] Nazari S, Salvi S, Visconti E, Caramella F, Rossi C, Rescigno G, Banfi C and Buniva P. (1999) Descending aorta substitution using a prosthesis with expandable ends. Case report. *J. Cardiovasc. Surg. (Torino)* 40: 417–420.

[30] Nazari S, Thoracic Aorta Substitution in less than 2 minutes. (2006)Video, *Proceedings 16th World Congress of World Society of Cardio- Thoracic Surgeons*, Ottawa, August 17-20, 2006.

[31] Nazari S. (2009) Modified Expandable Device for Easy and Realiable Dissection Layers Approximation in Sutureless Aortic Anastomosis. Video, *proceedings of The Houston Aortic Symposium*, Houston, March 26-28, 2009.

[32] Nazari S (2010) Expandable device type III for easy and reliable approximation of dissection layers in sutureless aortic anastomosis. Ex vivo experimental study. *Interact. CardioVasc. Thorac. Surg.* 10:161-164; originally published online Nov 20, 2009; DOI: 10.1510/icvts.2009. 216291.

[33] Parodi JC, Palmaz JC and Barone HD (1991) Transfemoral intraluminal graft implantation for abdominal aortic aneurysms. *Ann. Vasc. Surg.* 5:491-9.

[34] Parodi JC. (1994) Endovascular repair of abdominal aortic aneurysms and other arterial lesions. *Surg. Technol. Int.* 3:431-6.

[35] Payr E. (1900) Beitrage zur Technik der Blutgefass und Nervennaht nebst Mittheilungentiber die Verwendung eines resorbierbaren Metalles in der Chirurgie. *Arch. Klin. Chir.;* 62:67–93.

[36] Rossella C, Rescigno G, Nazari S. (2008) Modified expandable device for easy, quick and blood-tight sutureless anastomosis in ascending aorta. *Proceedings of The Houston Aortic Symposium*, April 2008.

[37] Ruby BJ and Cogbill TH (2007) Aortoduodenal fistula 5 years after endovascular abdominalaortic aneurysm repair with the Ancure stent graft. *J. Vasc. Surg.* 45:834-6.

[38] Schermerhorn ML, O'Malley AJ, Jhaveri A, Cotterill P, Pomposelli F, Landon BE. (2008) Endovascular vs. open repair of abdominal aortic aneurysms in the Medicare population. *N. Engl. J. Med.* 2008; 358: 464–474.

[39] Takata M, Watanabe G, Ohtake H, Ushijima T, Yamaguchi S, Kikuchi Y and Yamamoto Y(2011): Automatic aortic anastomosis with an innovative computer-controlled circular stapler for surgical treatment of aortic aneurysm. *J. Thorac. Cardiovasc. Surg.* 141:1265-9.

[40] Tanaka S, Kameda N, Kubo Y, Obatake N, Wakasa T, Ohsawa M and Wakasa K. (2009) Secondary aortoduodenal fistula caused on the suture line of the wrapping. *Pathology International* 59: 598–600 doi:10.1111/j.1440-1827.2009.02414.x.

[41] Tsagakis K, Pacini, D, Di Bartolomeo R et al. (2011).: Arch replacement and downstream stent grafting in complex aortic dissection: first results of an international registry. *Eur. J. CardioThor. Surg.* 39:87-94.

[42] Tesauro B. (1967) Impiego degli adesivi plastici e delle cucitrici meccaniche in chirurgia vascolare. Atti del 698 Congresso della Societa` Italiana di Chirurgia, Firenze 18– 20 Ottobre 1967. In: Fegiz G, editor. *Archivio ed atti della Societ`a Italiana di Chirurgia*. Roma: EMES, 1:663–790.

[43] Tesauro B and Persico G. (1979) Valutazione critica delle suture meccaniche in chirurgia vascolare. Atti dell'818 Congresso della Societa` Italiana di Chirurgia, Catania 8–11 Ottobre 1979. In: Fegiz G, editor. *Archivio ed atti della Società Italiana di Chirurgia*, Bologna: CLUEB, 1:633– 652.

[44] The UK EVAR Trial Investigators, Greenhalgh RM, Brown LC, Powell JT, Thompson SG, Epstein D, Sculpher MJ.(2010) Endovascular versus open repair of abdominal aortic aneurysm. *N. Engl. J. Med.* 2010; 362: 1863–1871.

[45] Wright KC, Wallace S, Charnsangavej C, Carrasco CH and Gianturco C (1985) Percutaneous endovascular stents: an experimental evaluation. *Radiology*. 156:69-72.

[46] Yoshioka T, Wright KC, Wallace S, Lawrence DD Jr and Gianturco C.(1988) Self-expanding endovascular graft: an experimental study in dogs. *AJR Am. J. Roentgenol.* 151:673-6.

[47] Zannini G (1967) Introduzione storica. In Atti del 69° Congresso della Societa` Italiana di Chirurgia, Firenze 18–20 Ottobre 1967. In: Fegiz G, editor. *Archivio ed atti della Società Italiana di Chirurgia*. Roma: EMES, 1:7-32.

In: Anastomoses ISBN: 978-1-62618-657-6
Editors: F. King, McKineley A. Malloy © 2013 Nova Science Publishers, Inc.

Chapter V

Bowel Anastomosis: Types, Techniques/Procedures, Clinical Outcomes and Complications

Jair Santos-Torres, Jaime Ruiz-Tovar, Antonio Arroyo and Rafael Calpena
General University Hospital of Elche,
Department of General and Digestive Surgery,
Elche, Alicante, Spain

Abstract

Despite development of improved surgical techniques, advances in perioperative and critical care and introduction of broad-spectrum antibiotics, colorectal surgery continues to present with as a great challenge. Postoperative complications are common, occurring in 18-57% of patients after elective surgery and in 39.3-72% after emergency one. Potential postoperative complications associated with the colorrectal surgery are complications related to anastomosis.

There is nothing that provokes greater anxiety and consternation to the gastrointestinal surgeon than the prospect of a leak from a colonic or colorectal anastomosis. The consequences to the patient from such a complication can be significant and not infrequently life-threatening. A surgeon can only control some of the many variables in anastomotic construction. The fundamental principles of preservation of an adequate blood supply, total absence of tension on the suture line and healthy bowel for both the proximal and distal ends without thickening or inflammation have remained constant. The necessity of bowel preparation is now a topic of considerable debate, defending many surgeons not to be performed. The technical requirements include the creation of an airtight suture line, in some circumstances protected by a proximal diverting procedure, and/or omental wrap. Whether the anastomosis is hand-sewn in one or two layers, performed with interrupted or running suture technique, or constructed with a stapling device has no impact on leak rates. Factors often beyond the surgeon's control are immutable comorbidities and the patient's body habitus.

A safe anastomosis should include: not leak, cause no persistent bleeding, cause no stricture of the lumen and create no risk for internal hernia. An ideal anastomosis must be also easy to construct, consistently reproducible, and easy to teach.

The aim of paper is to review types, techniques, procedures, clinical outcomes and complications of colorectal anastomoses, including mechanical and hand-sewn sutures, of the colonic and colorectal anastomoses. We expect to help surgeons and surgical fellows to learn about this topic with particular attention to the risk factors and procedure-related complications.

Introduction

Despite the development of improved surgical techniques, advances in perioperative and critical care and introduction of broad-spectrum antibiotics, colorectal surgery continues presenting with as a great challenge. Postoperative complications are common, occurring in 18-57% of patients after elective surgery and in 39.3-72% after emergency colorectal surgery. A number of prospective studies, both multicenter and single center, have evaluated patient outcomes after colorectal surgery. The rate of major morbidity ranged from 20 to 35% and the 30-day mortality rate ranged from 2 to 9 %. Potential postoperative complications associated with the colorrectal surgery are complications related to anastomosis. This may be secondary to ischemia, bleeding, leakage and inappropriate technique (i.e. inadequate tissue approximation) [1-5].

Options for restoring bowel continuity after a resection include an end-to-end, side-to-end or side-to-side colorectal, colocolic or ileocolic anastomosis, which can be either performed with a stapling device or hand-sewn. Stapled anastomosis requires less time to be performed and offers the potential for reduced fecal contamination. An alternative anastomosis that can be used between the proximal and distal colon (not rectum) is the functional end-to-end anastomosis, which is technically a side-to-side approach. There is insufficient evidence that any configuration is better functionally or less likely to leak, or that a stapled colorectal anastomosis is superior to a hand-sewn in ileocolic and colocolic anastomosis; the decision is based upon surgeon experience, preference, and available equipment [6-8]. However, in colorectal anastomosis, specially referring to lower rectal resections, though there is no enough evidence of better results with stapled devices, some trials show better result with this approach due to technical difficulty of the hand-sewn procedures [9-10].

Over the past two decades, numerous different materials have been used to join one bowel end to the other one, including catgut, stainless steel and newer monofilamentous and absorbable sutures. In the past 30 years, stapling devices have been embraced enthusiastically by the surgical community. The diffusion in the 80' decade of the stapler has modified the habits of the surgeons and the possibility to operate cancer of lower rectum, but leaving unchanged the rates of postoperative complications and bringing to the footlights some new complications. However, the choice of either technique in fashioning anastomosis is a matter of controversy among various schools [10].

The aim of paper is to review types, techniques, procedures, clinical outcomes and complications of colorectal anastomoses, including mechanical and hand-sewn sutures, of the colonic and colorectal anastomoses. We expect to help surgeons and surgical fellows to learn about this topic with particular attention to the risk factors and procedure-related complications.

Broadly speaking, there are three methods in the bowel anastomosis using a single-layer hand sewn suture: (a) An end-to-end anastomosis can be used when bowel ends are of similar diameter. (b) An end-to-side anastomosis can be used when the proximal end presents a wider diameter than the distal end, e.g. in small bowel obstruction. (c) A side-to-end anastomosis can be used when the distal end is greater in diameter than the proximal end, e.g. in right hemicolectomy. Anyway, the election of each technique depends on the surgeons' preferences. Figure 1.

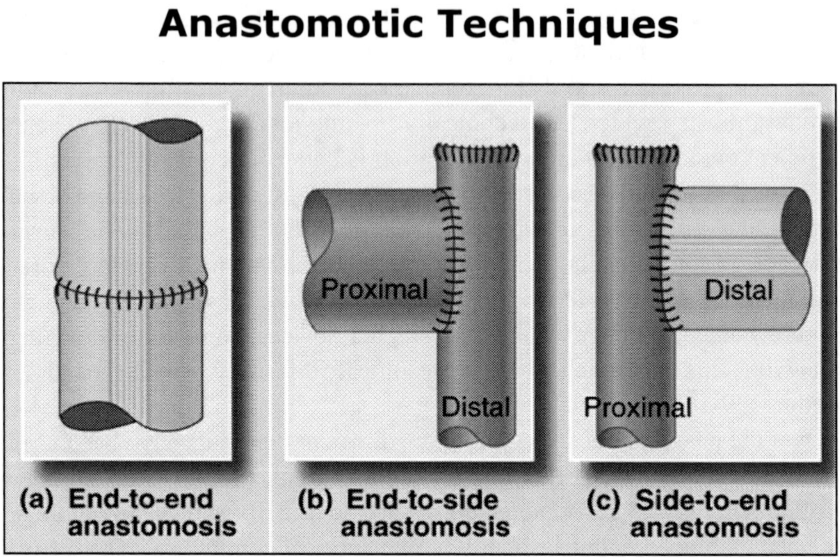

Figure 1. Methods of matching the diameter of the bowel ends to effect a safe anastomosis. *Source*: modified from reference [11].

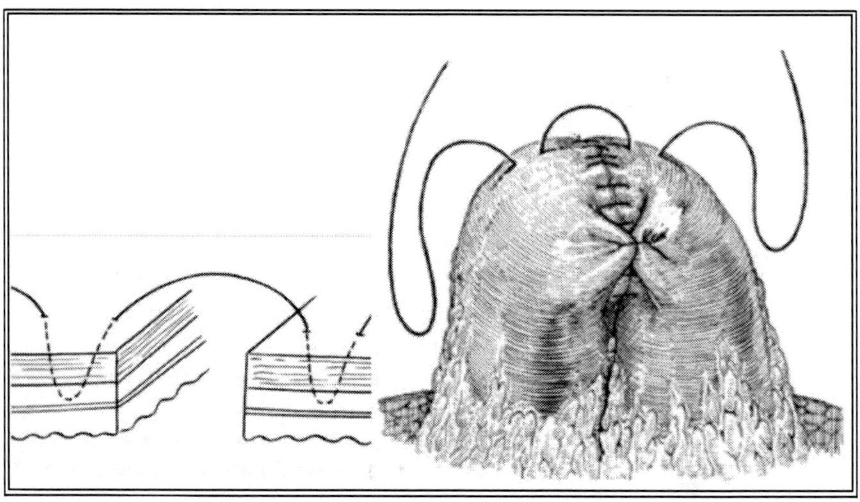

Figure 2. Lember sutures.

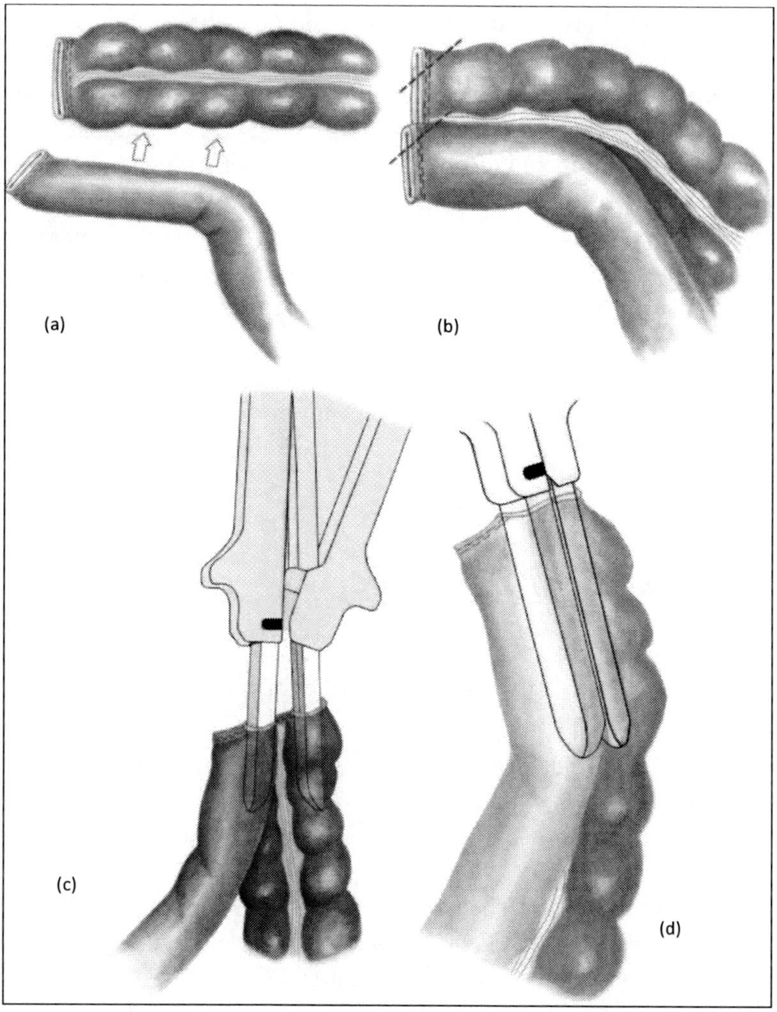

Figure 3. Side-to-side (functional end to end) anastomosis. *Source*: from reference [12].

Side to Side Anastomosis (Functional End to End Anastomosis): Using a Stapler

This kind of anastomosis is frequently used in open right colon resection. In this case, after the division of the bowel using a GIA 80 mm stapler, the ileum and transverse colon are aligned side-to-side (a). The antimesenteric corners of the bowel are cut off just before the GIA 80 mm stapler (GIA 80 mm stapler, United States Surgical Corp.) (b). The bowel ends are aligned and the stapler tines are inserted without tension on either small or large intestines (c). The GIA 80 mm stapler is fired creating a side-to-side (functional end to end) anastomosis. This technique is fast, and permits a wide union between the ileum and colon regardless of discrepancy of diameters of the two bowel ends. The remaining open section of intestine is closed either with a separate firing of a linear stapler (PI 55 mm, United States Surgical Corp.) or using a hand sewn technique of running 3/0 absorbable sutures. Some surgeons put several interrupted 3/0 absorbable “Lembert” sutures (Figure 2) into the crotch of the stapled anastomosis and any interesting staple lines. We prefer using a 80 mm stapler device rather than a shorter one, trying to obtain a wide anastomosis, avoiding future anastomotic strictures related with cicatricial fibrosis in some cases. Figure 3.

Side-to-Side Anastomosis: Hand Sewn

Anastomosis when the gut is of very different diameter and end to end or end to side anastomosis is difficult, as may happen if it is obstructed: (1) In the new- born when the distal gut is small, because it has never contained anything but meconium. (2) In older patients when end-to-end anastomosis is difficult because of differences in diameter. (3) When gut is difficult to mobilize because of adhesions, as sometimes when anastomosing the ileum to the colon.

If gut has to be resected, first close the ends of both loops of the gut to be anastomosed, as for the larger end of an end-to-side anastomosis described above (A, to G, Figure 4). If there is no gut to be resected, leave the ends in continuity.

Expel as much of the contents of both loops as you can, and apply non-crushing clamps about 6 cm from the ends of each. Insert a posterior layer of interrupted Lembert sutures or a running one including the seromuscular coats of both of them, starting with stay sutures at each end about 1 cm from the line of your proposed incision (A, in Figure 4).

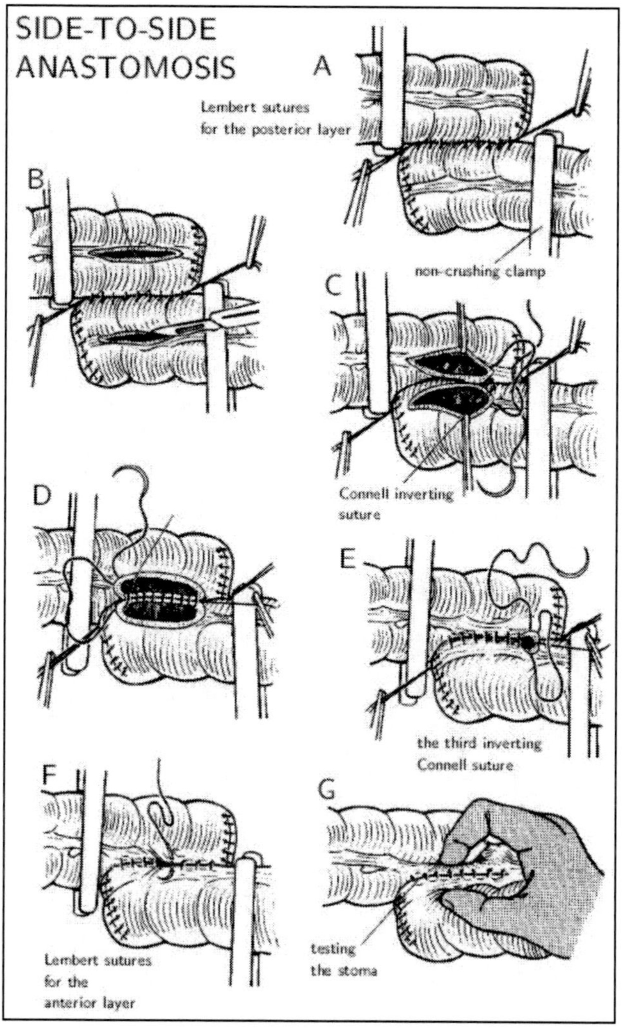

Figure 4. Site-to-site anastomosis: hand sewn. A, if, as in this figure, gut has been resected, close the ends of the two pieces of gut as in the previous figure. If, as is usually the case, and you are merely doing a bypass operation, no gut has been resected, leave the ends in continuity. Hold them with stay sutures and join them with the Lembert sutures that will form the posterior layer of the anastomosis. B, open both pieces of gut. C, start the posterior all-coats layer with a Connell stitch. D, the posterior all coats layer has reached the other end, so now insert another Connell stitch. E, the third and final Connell stitch. F, insert the anterior Lembert layer. G, test the stoma for patency. *Source*: from reference [13].

Incise both pieces of gut for about 3 cm, in the line of a taenia in the case of the colon (B). Starting with a Connell inverting stitch (C), use 2/0 or 3/0 (depending on the bowel wall thickness) absorbable suture to join the posterior cut edges of the gut with an all coats continuous over-and-over suture (D). When you reach the other end make another Connell inverting stitch. Then continue the over-and-over continuous suture along the anterior layer of the anastomosis. Finally, complete it with another Connell inverting stitch (E) and tie the ends of the suture together, leaving 5 mm cut ends.

Insert an anterior layer of 2/0 or 3/0 absorbable Lembert or running seromuscular sutures (F). Test the lumen of the stoma with your fingers (G) and move the gut contents over the anastomosis to check for leaks.

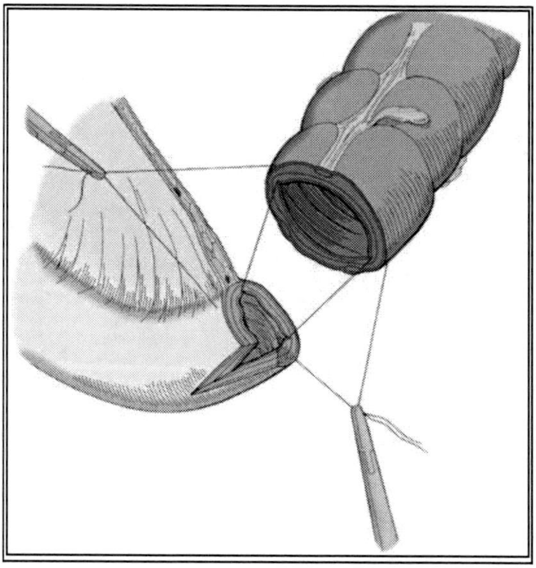

Figure 5. The single Cheatle slit. *Source*: modified from reference [14].

End-to-End Anastomosis: Hand Sewn (Figure 6)

A standard end-to-end anastomosis can be performed between two segments of small bowel, ileum and colon, or two segments of colon using a single layer of interrupted sutures. Absorbable sutures 3/0 (polyglycolic acid/polyglactin) with a tapered needle are frequently used. The discrepancy in size of the lumens between ileum and large intestine can be accommodated with a Cheatle slit on the antimesenteric side of the ileum for an end to end anastomosis. (Figure 5).

Stapled end-to-end anastomosis are most frequently used in colorectal anastomosis and are later on described.

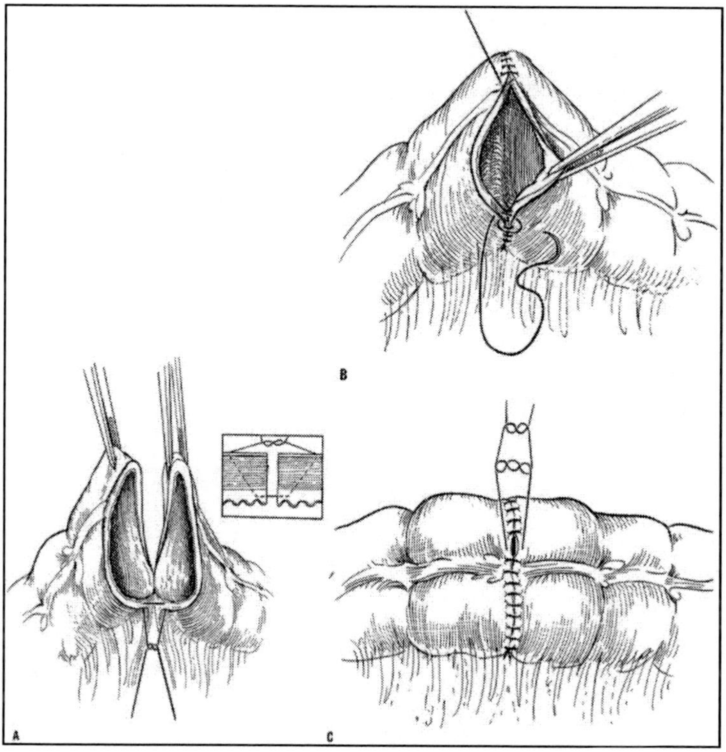

Figura 6. End-to-end anastomosis: hand sewn.

End-to-Side Anastomosis: Hand Sewn

An end-to-side anastomosis is commonly used in the operations of right hemicolectomy or subtotal colectomy. In an end-to-side anastomosis one segment of the bowel must be closed. To close the bowel, a two-layer inverting suture technique can be used (stapled and inverting suture of the staple line); this technique could be done with a single-layer hand sewn suture. The bowel end is held in a non-crushing clamp and starting at the antimesenteric border a 3/0 absorbable suture is inserted as a continuous horizontal mattress suture. This is then tied at the mesenteric border and the stitch returned as a continouous over-and-over stitch incorporating the full thickness of the bowel wall. The described method is a single-layer suture; however, this anastomosis can also be performed as a two-layer technique. In this way, a first seromuscular suture of the posterior face of the anastomosis is performed from the mesenteric border to the antimesenteric one, followed by a full thickness suture of the posterior and anterior face of the anastomosis, similarly to the already described single-layer suture. Finally, in the two-layer anastomosis a continuous seromuscular suture of the anterior face of the anastomosis is performed invaginating the mucosa. Both layers are usually sutured with absorbable material that can be mono or polifilamentous. (Figure 7).

Some studies show that two-layer intestinal anastomosis offers no definite advantage over single-layer anastomosis in terms of postoperative leak. Considering duration of the anastomosis procedure and medical expenses, some authors defend single-layer intestinal anastomosis as the optimal choice in most surgical situations [15].

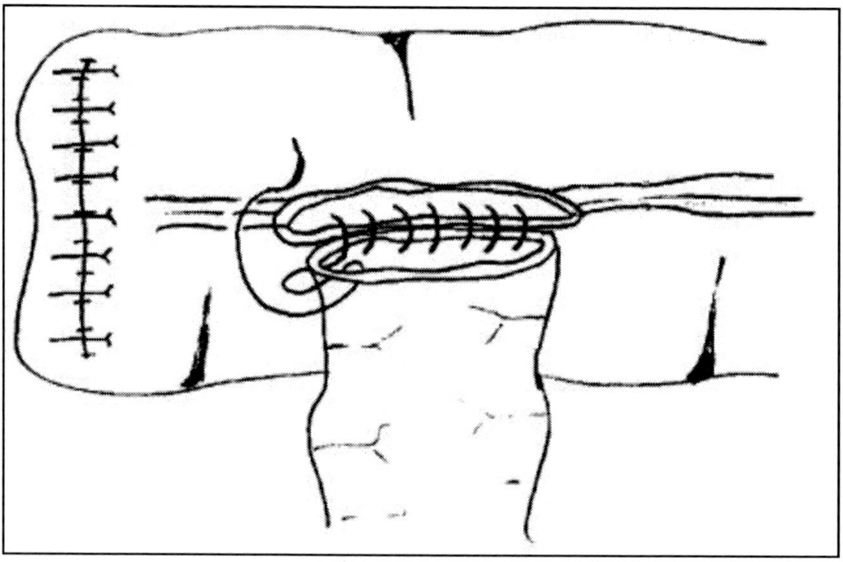

Figure 7. End-to-side anastomosis: hand sewn.

Two layered technique is the classic teaching of GastroIntestinal (GI) anastomosis. This technique produced serosal apposition and mucosal inversion, and the inner layer believed to be haemostatic but also strangulates mucosa. The single layered technique is the modern teaching of GI anastomoses. This technique incorporates strong submucosal layer and minimal damage to submucosal vascular plexus.

Colorectal Anastomosis

For colorectal or coloanal anastomoses, there are essentially six technical alternatives:

1. Hand-sewn end to end
2. Circular stapled end to end
3. Circular stapled side to end
4. Circular stapled with colonic J-pouch

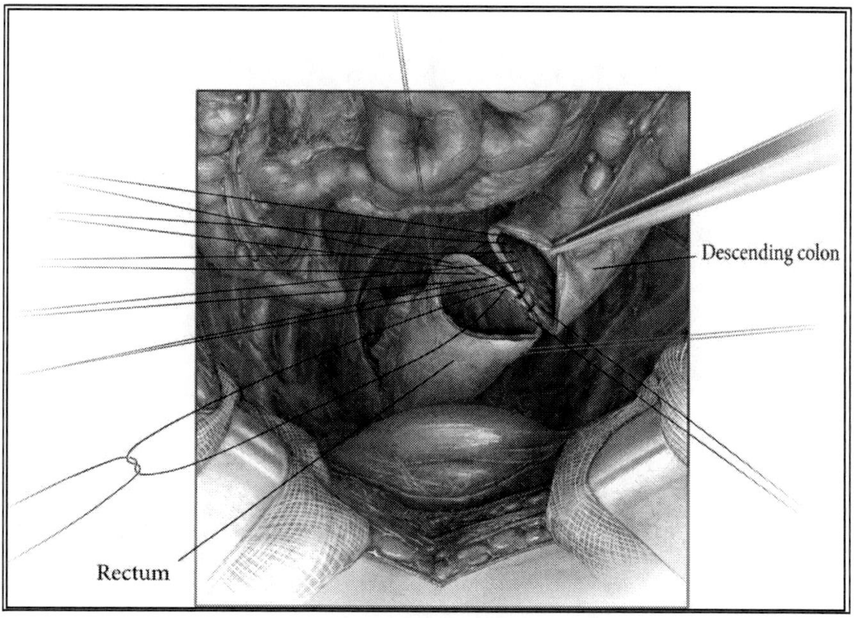

Figure 8. Hand-sewn anastomosis between the transected proximal colon and the rectum after sigmoid colectomy. *Source*: from reference [16].

The choice of a given anastomosis is to some degree at the discretion and preference of the surgeon, but also based on the level of transection of the rectum and the anatomy of the patient. Most anastomoses above 7 to 8 cm can be either hand sewn or stapled (Figs 8 and 9). In patients with a fatty mesenterium and/or short sigmoid vasculature, the side to end technique can provide a more comfortable reach of the sigmoid colon into the deep pelvis, and can reduce the amount of mesenteric mobilization required (Fig 10). It also allows the anastomosis to be made through the antimesenteric border of the sigmoid colon, which in an obese patient may be the only area free of significant attached fatty tissue. The suture line should be set up to be sure the distal aspect of the anastomosis is 1 cm. proximal to the closed sigmoid end. For the coloanal anastomosis, the dissection to remove the rectum is the same whether the anastomosis is hand-sewn or stapled.

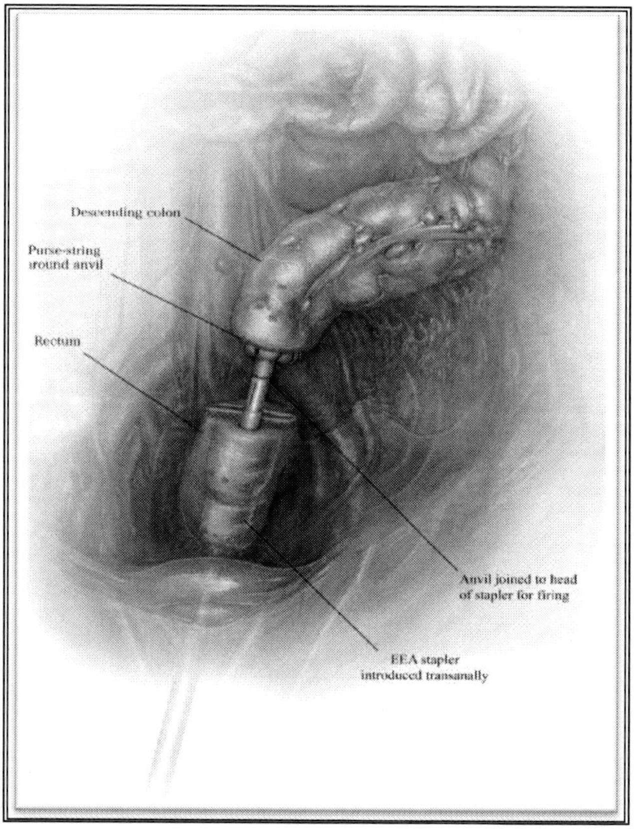

Figure 9. End-to-end anastomosis (EEA) with the circular stapler, joining the transected proximal colon to the rectum after sigmoid colectomy. *Source*: from reference [13].

The hand-sewn alternative in coloanal anastomosis requires a transanal approach for placing the sutures, and is performed in a single layer (Fig 11). The stapled alternative can either be a straight coloanal approach, or incorporate the use of a small colonic J-pouch (Fig 12A and B).

There are other decisions the surgeon has to make once the anastomosis has been constructed: Whether to perform a temporary diverting stoma and which type of stoma this should be, the placement of drains, and the reinforcement of the anastomosis with an omental flap. There is a significant consensus that routine diversion is indicated in all coloanal anastomoses, as these carry the highest leak rate (10-15%).

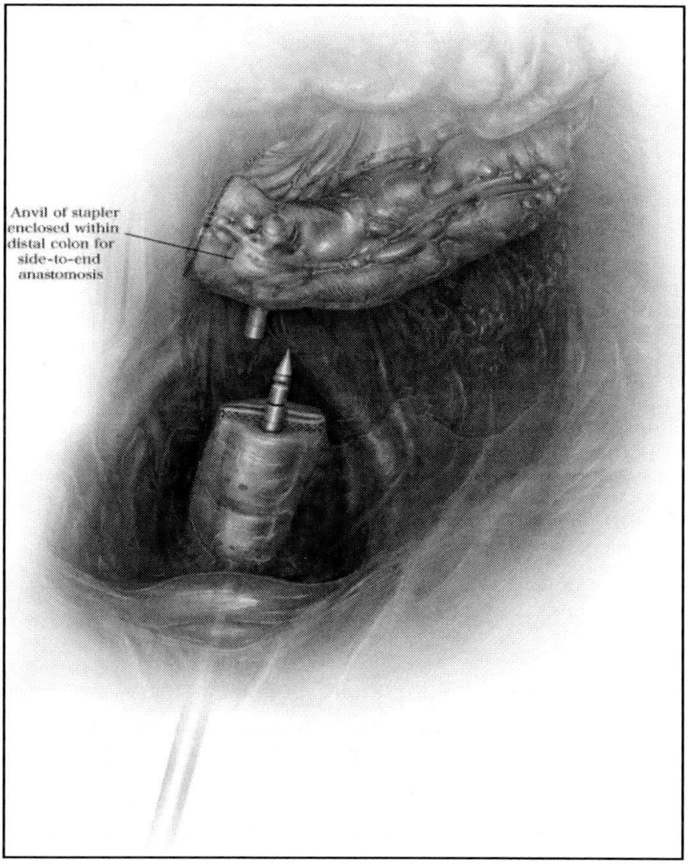

Figure 10. Anastomosis joining the side of the transected colon to the end of the transected rectum after sigmoid colectomy. *Source*: from reference [16].

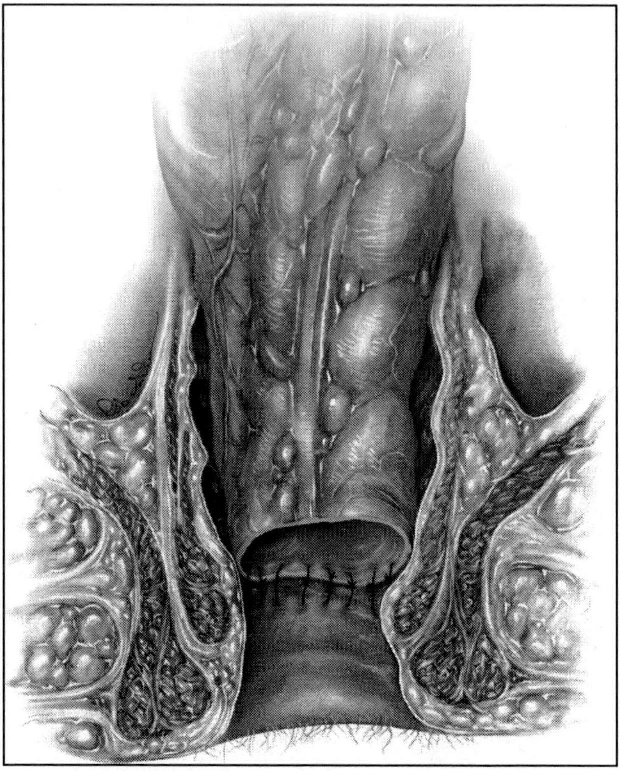

Figure 11. Single layer hand-sewn transanal anastomosis of colon to anus. *Source*: from reference [16].

Since these low anastomoses can very rarely be revised or redone, a coloanal reconstruction is essentially a "one shot" endeavor; all reasonable measures to protect it are warranted. Most surgeons would also agree that temporary diversion is reasonable for any anastomosis at or below 7 to 8 cm, or when preoperative radiation therapy was administered. Diversion can be accomplished with either a proximal loop colostomy or ileostomy. A temporary loop ileostomy has the advantage of being easily delivered through the abdominal wall, and being straightforward to close, usually through a peri-stomal approach. This saves the patient from having a second major laparotomy incision, and is typically a brief procedure with a short hospital stay. Several recent studies have also demonstrated that a loop ileostomy accomplishes essentially 100% fecal diversion. The long length of defunctionalized colon has never been shown to generate an adverse outcome [17].

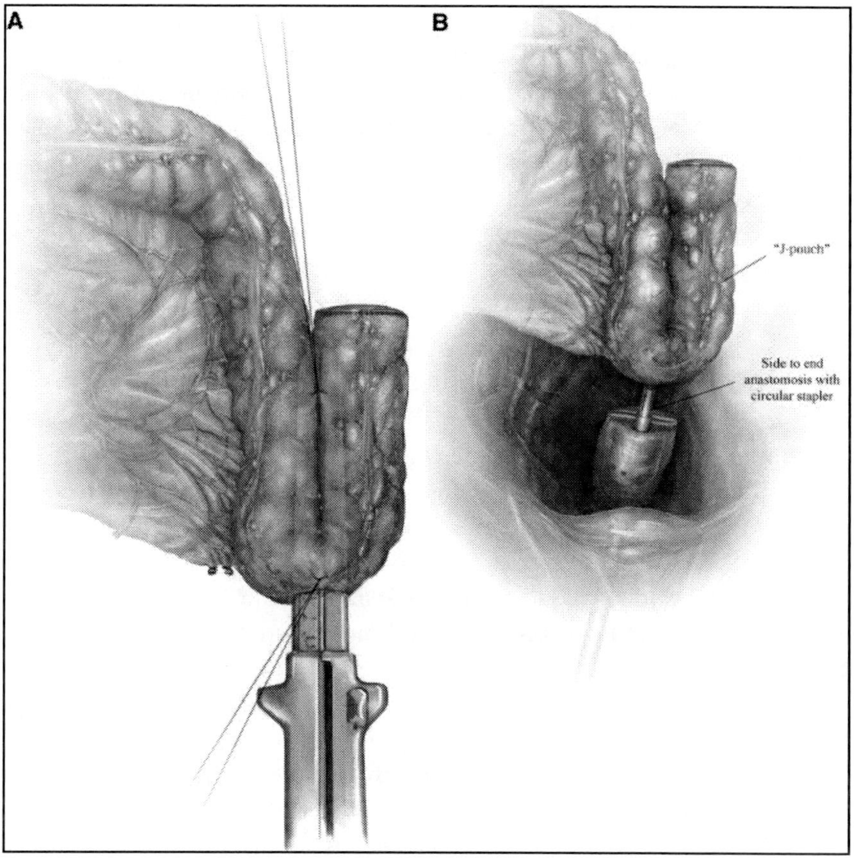

Figure 12. (A) J pouch coloanal anastomosis. The linear stapler is used to create a reservoir in the previously mobilized colon. (B) J pouch coloanal anastomosis. On removal of the lineal stapler, the circular stapler is introducer through the rectum and intocolostomy, where a side-to-end anastomosis is created between colon and rectum. *Source*: from reference [16].

The use of pelvic drains has been shown in most studies to either have no benefit or to actually increase the incidence of leaks. Nevertheless, most surgeons are understandably uncomfortable with the notion of significant fluid and debris accumulation in the dependent pelvis after a very low or coloanal reconstruction, and the specific circumstances of the individual procedure should determine whether drains are used or not. If the operation is technically difficult and/or generates significant blood loss or oozing, a drain may be reasonably used [18].

Employing an omental wrap around an anastomosis in the pelvis carries a common sense appeal, provided there is sufficient omentum to reach the pelvis. This is usually accomplished by creating an omental pedicle off of either the right or left gastroepiploic arcade. The limited clinical studies assessing this maneuver have shown results similar to what is accomplished with a proximal diversion; the leak rate is not significantly reduced, but the omental wrap confines the leak to the pelvis and diminishes the likelihood of a more widespread peritonitis [19].

Colorectal Anastomotic Complications

Failure of an anastomosis with leakage of intestinal contents is one of the most significant surgical complications. Reported leakage rates range from 4 to 26%, depending on what type of anastomosis was performed and whether the operation was an elective or an emergency procedure. An anastomotic leak increases the morbidity and mortality associated with the operation: it can double the length of the hospital stay and increase the mortality as much as 10fold [20-21].

Signs and symptoms suggestive of an anastomotic leak include postoperative (usually between days 4 to 7) abdominal pain or peritonitis, fever, leukocytosis, elevation of de C-reactive protein and procalcitonin. An abdominal X -ray showing free air or a CT scan with pneumoperitoneum and significant free fluid or inflammatory changes around the anastomosis are suggestive of an anastomotic leak. In the lower anastomosis of colon and rectum, it is useful to perform an anal contrast-enhanced CT scan for a more reliable diagnosis of the leakage.

A localized anastomotic leak that is not associated with peritonitis or significant systemic sepsis can be managed with percutaneous or open drainage of the abscess, however anastomotic leaks associated with peritonitis or systemic manifestation of sepsis require a laparotomy and either revision of the anastomosis if feasible or fecal diversion proximally or at the site of the anastomosis.

Factors Contributing to Anastomotic Failure

Type and Location

As a rule, for any given technique the location of the anastomosis does not influence the overall leakage rate. There are two exceptions to this general rule. First, low anterior rectal and ultra-low anterior anastomosis are associated with leakage rates ranging from 4.5% to 8%, however an acceptable leak rate is around 5% [22].

Bowel Preparation

For elective anastomoses of the colon and rectum, it is traditional to cleanse the large bowel prior to surgery. The rationale being that decreasing the bacterial load in the colon facilitates anastomotic healing and decreases the incidence and consequences of anastomotic leakage, is nowadays a controversial issue. Recent studies have questioned this approach and there is increasing evidence that a bowel preparation may not be essential and that it may actually have even some disadvantages [23].

Associated Diseases and Systemic Factors

Age, infection, hypotension and hypoperfusion states, intraoperative transfusion, carcinoma at the line of reception, anemia, diabetes mellitus, previous irradiation or chemotherapy, malnutrition with hypoalbuminemia, vitamin deficiencies, chronic steroid use, smoking, and certain disease conditions, like Crohn's disease, are associated with poor anastomotic healing and increased anastomotic leak rates.

In spite of the fact that leakage cannot be entirely prevented, principles of good technique must be observed:

- Anastomose only healthy colon
- Avoid tension on the anastomosis
- Ensure a good blood supply at the cut ends of both bowels. Good color, bleeding at the cut edge, and pulsation of mesenteric vessels are indicators of a good blood supply.
- Avoid intramural hematoma. If a hematoma appears to be spreading, do not hesitate to resect more colon. Good hemostasis is absolutely mandatory; ligate all vessels.
- Clean fat, epiploic appendices, and mesentery from both proximal and distal edges of the anastomosis. Clean not more than 1 to 1.5 cm.

Ensure that these maneuvers do not compromise the blood supply to the bowel ends.

- Preserve an adequate lumen
- Close mesenteric gaps if possible. If they cannot be closed, open them as wide as possible to avoid postoperative internal hernias.
- Adequate preioperative antibiotic systemic prophylaxis is mandatory.
- If there is any doubt about the correct performance of the anastomosis, do a proximal colostomy. This is a life-saving procedure.

Anastomotic Bleeding

Anastomotic bleeding is common, varies in severity. In most cases, bleeding is minor and is manifested by the passage of dark blood with the patient's first bowel movements after surgery. It is related to the choice of surgical approach, location of anastomosis and in rectal surgery with or without preventive colostomy. Some studies have shown that laparoscopic surgery is a risk factor, and preventive colostomy is a protective factor in rectal surgery. Most cases are mild and self-limited. More serious bleeding, especially that from colonic or ileal pouches, can be successfully managed with epinephrine (1:100,000) and saline retention enemas. If this fails, or bleeding is massive and results in hemodynamic instability, the patient is best returned to the operating room for surgical intervention. In cases of bleeding small bowel or proximal colonic anastomoses, angiography with selective infusion of vasopressin or embolization of the bleeding vessel may be indicated [24, 25].

Anastomotic Strictures

Anastomotic stricture may be the end result of anastomotic leak or ischemia. It typically presents 2–12 months after surgery with increasing constipation and difficulty evacuating. If the initial resection was done for malignancy, recurrence as a cause of the stricture must be excluded with a combination of CT scan and fluorodeoxyglucose–positron emission tomography (PET) scan. Biopsy is mandatory if a mass or abnormality is identified. Low colorectal, coloanal, or ileal pouch-anal anastomotic strictures may be successfully treated with repeated dilations using an examining finger or rubber dilators. Dilation is more successful if initiated within the first few weeks after surgery. In fact, almost all coloanal or ileoanal anastomoses will stricture to some degree during the early postoperative period, especially if a diverting stoma is present. All such anastomoses should undergo digital examination at 4–6 weeks after surgery and just before stoma closure (usually at 2–3 months). Strictures are usually soft and easily dilated during these examinations. Higher colorectal, colocolic or ileocolic strictures may be approached using endoscopic balloon dilation. If these measures fail, or if the stricture is extremely tight or long, revision surgery may be required. These are difficult operations, however, because of the pelvic fibrosis that develops after anastomotic leak and complications are common. In some cases, permanent fecal diversion is the only option [24-27].

Early obstruction at the anastomotic site can result from edema or excessive inversion; late obstruction can be caused by recurrent carcinoma.

References

[1] Slieker JC, Komen N, Komen NA, et al. Long-term and perioperative corticosteroids in anastomotic leakage: a prospective study of 259 left-sided colorectal anastomoses. *Arch Surg*. 2012; 147:447-52.

[2] Alves A, Panis Y, Mathieu P, et al. Postoperative mortality and morbidity in French patients undergoing colorectal surgery: results of a prospective multicenter study. *Arch Surg*. 2005; 140:278-83.

[3] Fazio VW, Tekkis PP, Remzi F, Lavery IC. Assessment of operative risk

[4] Tekkis PP, Poloniecki JD, Thompson MR

[5] Ho YH, Ashour MA. Techniques for colorectal anastomosis. *World J Gastroeneterol* 2010; 16:1610-21.

[6] Neutzling CB, Lutosa SA, Proenca IM, et al. Stapled versus handsewn methods for colorectal anastomosis surgery. *Cochrane Databased of Systematic Reviews* 2012; (2):CD003144.

[7] Leung E, Ferjani AM, Stellard N, Wong LS. Predicting post-operative mortality

[8] Ruiz-Tovar J, Santos J, Arroyo A, et al. Microbiological spectrum of the intraperitoneal surface after elective right-sided colon cancer: are there differences in the peritoneal contamination after performing a stapled or a handsewn anastomosis?. *Int J Colorectal Dis* 2012; 27:1515-9.

[9] Ishii Y, Hasegawa H, Nishibori H, et al. The application of a new stapling device for open surgery (Contour TM Curved Cutter Stapler) in

the laparoscopic resection of the rectal cancer. *Surg Endosc* 2006; 20:1329-31.

[10] Neutzling CB, Lustosa SA, Proencia IM, et al. Stapled versus handsewn methods for colorectal anastomosis surgery. *Cochrane Database sys Rev* 2012; 15;2CD003144.

[11] Elseiver. Burkitt et al: Essential Surgery 4e – *www.studentconsult.com*

[12] Milson JW. Hunt D. Open right colon resection. *Operative Techniques in General Surgery* 2003; 5:190-8.

[13] *http://ps.cnis.ca/wiki/index.php/Methods_for_abdominal_surgery*

[14] The McGraw-Hill Companies. Skandalakis J. et al: *Skandalakis' Surgical Anatomy*

[15] Shikata S, Yamagishi H, Taji Y, et al. Single- versus two-layer intestinal anastomosis: meta-analysis of randomized control trials. *BMC Surgery* 2006;6:2.

[16] Stahl T. Technical considerations in the difficult colorectal anastomosis. *Operative Techniques in General Surgery* 2007; 9:139-84.

[17] Marusch F, Kock A, Schmidt U, et al. Value of a protective stoma in low anterior resections for rectal cancer. *Dis Colon Rectum* 2002; 45:1164-71.

[18] Karliczek A, Jesus EC, Matos D, et al. Drainage or nondrainage in elective colorectal anastomosis: a systematic review and meta-analysis. *Colorectal Dis* 2006; 8:259-65.

[19] Agnifili A, Schietroma M, Carloni A, et al. The value of omentoplasty in protecting colorectal anastomosis from leakage. A prospective randomized study in 126 patients. *Hepatogastroenterology* 2004; 51:1694-7.

[20] Boccola MA, Lin J, Rozen WN, et al. Reducing anastomotic leakage in oncologic colorectal surgery: an evidence- based review. *Anticancer Res* 2010; 30:601-7.

[21] Platell C, Barwood N, Dorfmann G, et al. The incidence of anastomotic leaks in patients undergoing colorectal surgery. *Colorectal Dis* 2007; 9:71-9.

[22] Buchs NC, Gervaz P, Secic M, et al. Incidence, consequences, and risk factors for anastomotic dehiscence after colorectal surgery: a prospective monocentric study. *Int J Colorectal Dis* 2008; 23:265-70.

[23] Cao F, Li J, Li F. Mechanical bowel preparation for elective colorectal surgery: updated systematic review and meta-analysis. *Int J Colorectal Dis* 2012; 27:803-10.

[24] Davis B, Rivadeneira DE. Complications of colorectal anastomoses: leaks, strictures, and bleeding. *Surg Clin North Am* 2013; 93:61-87.

[25] Dietz DW. Postoperative complications. In*: The ASCRS textbook of colon and rectal surgery*, Wolff BG, Fleshman JW, Beck DE, et al. New York, Springer Science +Business Media, 2011:pp 141-55.

[26] Di Giorgio P, De Luca L, Rivellini G, et al. Endoscopic dilation of benign colorectal anastomotic stricture after low anterior resection: a prospective comparison study of two balloon types. *Gastrointest Endosc* 2004; 60:347–50.

[27] Suchan KL, Muldner A, Manegold BC. Endoscopic treatment of postoperative colorectal anastomotic strictures. *Surg Endosc* 2003; 17:1110–13.

Index

C

D

H

I

N

O

P

Q

R

S

T

U

V

W